Dr. Knee

A Surgeon's Alternative to Knee Replacement

By Shaw-Ruey Lyu, MD, PhD

Copyright © 2016 Shaw-Ruey Lyu

All rights reserved.

ISBN-10: 1530021642
ISBN-13: 978-1530021642

*This book is dedicated to all
who accompany, cherish, and enlighten me
through my lonely pursuits,
past, present, and future.*

Preface 5

Chapter 1 Terminology 18

Chapter 2 The KHPO in A Nutshell 24

Chapter 3 What Has ACRFP Done for Patients? It Has Helped Their Cartilage Regrow 41

Chapter 4 The Hidden Hazards of Ineffective Conservative Treatments 49

Chapter 5 Why is the ACRFP Better for the Knees? Its Distinctions and Advantages 60

Chapter 6 Knee OA Treatments: The Conventional Protocol vs the KHPO Protocol 70

Chapter 7 Patient Activism 82

Chapter 8 A Concerned Surgeon and His Thoughts 86

Chapter 9 Evidence-based Medicine Part I: Patients' Choices . 90

Chapter 10 Evidence-Based Medicine Part II: Physician's Clinical Experiences 113

Chapter 11 Evidence-Based Medicine Part III: The Best Scientific Evidence 126

Chapter 12 The Making of an Ideal KHPO Surgeon 133

Appendix 1:   She helps make ACRFP work so well 139

Appendix 2:   The three rehabilitation exercises under the KHPO 147

Appendix 3:   Activities to enjoy or to avoid before and during the first post-operative year of ACRFP 151

Biography 152

ACKNOWLEDGMENTS

This book was made possible through the outstanding contributions of many individuals. My colleagues at the Knee Health Promotion Centre of Tzu-Chi Medical Foundation interviewed, collected, and organised all the fundamental clinical data for the book. I extend my special appreciation to all the patients and KHPO fellows who share their experiences as testimonials. The making of this book would have been impossible without the efforts of our research team (listed in Chapter 11), to whom I owe my sincere gratitude.

I am most grateful to Mr. Yau-Yang Tang for his work in translating and editing this book. His enthusiasm and talent for conceptualisation were invaluable in finalising the contents and design of the book.

To all who helped, I would like to say again, thank you very much.

Shaw-Ruey Lyu

Preface

Scientia est potentia (Knowledge is power).

- Sir Francis Bacon, 1561-1626

Kept her knees for as long as she needed them

For her knee OA, Mrs. Lee could have received knee replacement from a superb surgeon, but instead she chose to keep her knees with the ACRFP under the KHPO, the subject matter of this book.

I operated on Mrs. Lee's knees in 2002 when she was 81. Her son, a professor of medicine, wrote in 2013, "It has been ten years since Dr. Lyu performed the ACRFP on my mother. Thanks to his treatment, my mother, now in her 90s, still walks around freely, independently, and without pain. She still enjoys herself. She and I would love to tell the world how wonderful the ACRFP has been for her."

She never received any artificial knees. Her own knees continued to serve her until she passed away in 2014. She was 93.

Likewise, thousands more of my patients have also kept their knees because I performed the ACRFP for them. I performed the ACRFP because I believed that it was the best treatment for them notwithstanding the fact that I like to perform another surgery more.

My favourite work as an orthopaedic surgeon has been knee replacement. I regularly perform knee replacements for around 300 patients annually, and I very much enjoy the tremendously positive feedback from my patients. However, I have gradually become somewhat reluctant to recommend it to my patients. Instead, when appropriate, I recommend something much better and much less invasive—the ACRFP.

Read on to find out. **Perhaps you may keep your knees and reclaim your life from knee osteoarthritis.**

Knee replacement is one of the most successful procedures in all of medicine. According to the Agency for Healthcare Research and Quality, more than 600,000 knee replacements are performed each year in the United States. While the success rate for knee replacement is quite high, a failure may lead to unmanageable suffering. The following two episodes led me to examine my practice, where I had successfully performed knee replacements for more than twenty years, and to find a cure that makes the seemingly unavoidable knee replacement operation unnecessary.

Episode 1

A farmer in his 70s had a total knee replacement (TKR) done elsewhere, but his prosthesis later became infected and purulent. He sought help from many doctors for two years to no avail, including several salvage operations. His purulent wounds required dressing several times a day, but still his infection was not cured.

Finally he came to see me in 2002, full of hope that I would give him a simple arthroscopy to cure his misery. However, his condition was too serious for that, and there was only one course of action left for him. I informed him that he would need two operations. The first operation would remove the infected artificial knee and implant antibiotics, which would be left in place for about three months, to kill off the bacteria. After the bacteria had been totally eliminated, the second operation would follow to put in another set of artificial knee (see Fig. 1 as an example).

Having already gone through many procedures including the ones I suggested and suffered so much without success, he did not want to try them again. However, he had come to see me too late, so I could not have offered him a less invasive option.

He rejected my recommendations and left my clinic disappointed.

My office called him three days later to follow up.

A neighbour of his told us that

the farmer had killed himself the day before!

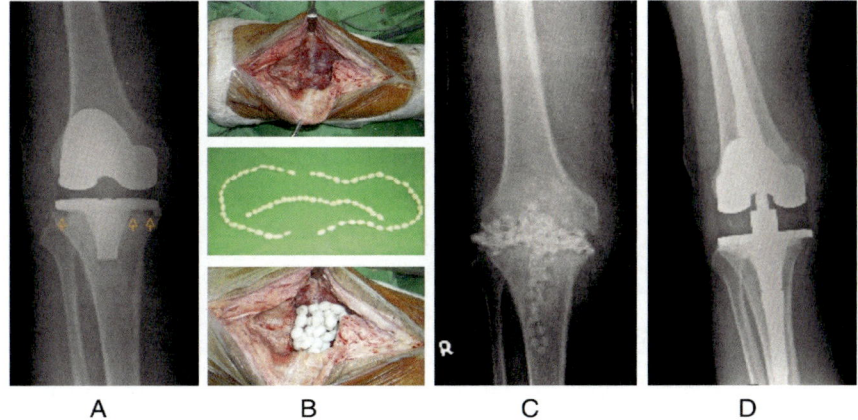

Fig. 1, (A) Three years after a successful total knee replacement surgery, this artificial knee is still infected by bacteria (the arrows mark the lesions). (B) The infected prosthesis is taken out, the infected tissues are thoroughly removed, and antibiotics are placed in the cavity. (C) The antibiotics are left in place for three months to totally eradicate the bacteria. (D) A new artificial knee is put in.

Statistically speaking, infections occur in 0.3 to 0.5 percent of TKR operations, even ones executed by a most experienced team in a best-equipped operating room. Even if a surgery is initially successful, bacterial infections are always lurking as long as an artificial knee is in a patient. Once a prosthesis is infected, a patient has just one option left (Fig. 1), the same two-operation option that I outlined for the farmer in 2002.

How can a patient not be very careful before choosing to have a knee replaced? How can a physician easily recommend a knee replacement without extra care and thought?

Episode 2

One autumn afternoon in 1995 a woman walked into my clinic. Her gaits gave her knee OA away. She seemed to know exactly what she wanted done about her knee OA. She wanted her knees replaced, and, based on the prevailing treatment guideline, I thought that she had a valid request. Furthermore, I did not know then what I know now.

I recommended knee replacement and requested approval from her insurance for total knee replacement, a process that would normally take four weeks.

As was customary in the local medical community then, I also recommended arthroscopy to give her temporary relief, which would last just a few months. She agreed to the procedure.

So we proceeded to the arthroscopy procedure. Deep in her knee I saw lesions that (1) I had never seen before and (2) had never been mentioned or described in literature before. I videotaped and took still photos of these lesions, and then, without an established treatment protocol to guide me, I instinctively started to thoroughly remove them. I saw many undocumented, unfamiliar images as I cleaned up her lesions. I was shocked because they were not in my knowledge base. The next day, the patient cheerfully thanked me because the knee pain that had dogged her for years was gone.

I discharged her that day, so she went home happy, and I returned to my practice all but forgetting about this episode because I did not realise at the time the significance of these hidden lesions.

Now, fast forward to one day in 2002. I had switched to my current hospital two years before. A throng of patients filled my clinic as usual.

That woman I operated on in 1995 cheerfully walked into my office. "Dr. Lyu, I'm here today *not* as a patient. I accidentally found that you are working here, and I just wanted to tell you that the arthroscopic treatment that you gave to my knee a few years back was great," she said. **My knee is cured. I've not needed medicine ever since the surgery.**"

Her words brought those hidden lesions back to life in my mind. She just told me that what I had done for her seven years before—removing the lesions and cleaning up the area—had **cured her knee OA**. That was a big deal!

Her reappearance and her words gave me a shot in the arm. Why would removing the hidden lesions and cleaning up the area relieve her knee pain, restore her knee function, and cure her degenerative knee? Was that a fluke or was there a cause-and-effect relationship? I decided to pursue the cause of knee OA. Again, this was 2002.

My pursuit has eventually led to a dozen research papers, the recognition of the terms "Medial Abrasion Syndrome (MAS)", the "Arthroscopic Medial Release (AMR)", the "Arthroscopic Cartilage Regeneration Facilitating Procedure" (ACRFP), the "Knee Health Promotion Option" (KHPO), and this book. More importantly, I have used these treatments to relieve thousands of knee OA sufferers of their debilitating pains.

A vast majority of them have kept their knees, have been pain-free, have regained function, and have resumed their lives, just as *that* **woman has.**

The conventional arthroscopic treatment vs the ACRFP for knee OA

The common conventional arthroscopic treatments for knee osteoarthritis (OA) include such procedures as arthroscopic lavage, debridement, chondroplasty, mosaicplasty, and resection of torn menisci. They are often considered ineffectual and over-utilised. I started practicing as an orthopaedic surgeon under this cook book approach in 1989. Having been in this camp for so long, I am fully aware of the capabilities and limitations of this treatment approach.

Our research team identified the pathogenesis of knee OA in 2004. Based on this research, I devised a novel procedure: the arthroscopic cartilage regeneration facilitating procedure (ACRFP), and I have switched to this approach ever since to treat knee OA because it is more effective than the conventional procedures.

The ACRFP is a comprehensive arthroscopic surgery that aims primarily to remove all existing risk factors from the knee, making the knee a more hospitable place for the cartilage inside to regenerate. In 2007, we further advanced and expanded this novel concept for treating knee OA to a multidisciplinary treatment protocol that we call knee health promotion option (KHPO) for the comprehensive management of this common disease. This book is about the KHPO.

Through this book, I hope to give patients of knee OA reason for hope, and I hope to offer a new, effective approach to cope with this disease that is as old as the human race (Fig. 2).

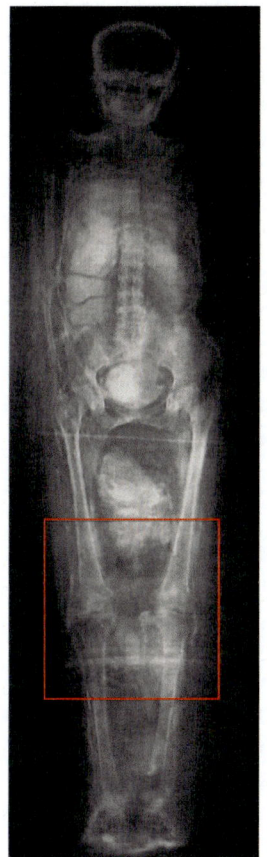 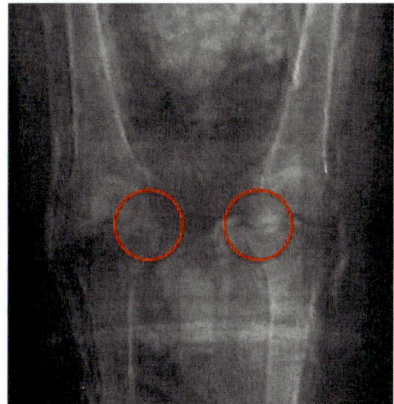

Fig. 2, A whole-body X-ray of a mummy at the British Museum shows stages II and III knee OA (the knee area enlarged, right).

The following comment from a patient of knee OA is quite typical in that it shows the pain, the helplessness, and the frustration that many patients of knee OA also experience.

My right knee hurt, and I started seeing doctors for it two years ago. I have seen doctors in many disciplines, such as orthopaedics, rheumatology, neurology, and family medicine. I have been through magnetic resonance imaging, nuclear scanning, whole body bone scanning, and many blood tests. All reports showed me as a normal, healthy person. It seems that all hospitals told me the same thing.

But still my knee hurts. I no longer know what doctors to see. The doctors know that I have knee pains, swelling, and oedema, but they do not know why my knee is repeatedly inflamed. All they can do is give me pain and anti-inflammatory drugs, which honestly do me no good.

I have tried traditional Chinese medicine. The thing was very expensive, but several months and a small fortune later, my knee still hurt. I tried acupuncture six days a week for a solid month, but that brought me no relief. I hurt every day, I could not sleep, and I took sleep aids. I could not work, so I had to shut down the clothing store that I had run for many years. I have stayed home because I cannot go anywhere without hurting. I shut myself out from the world, and I feel my future fading away.

In the last two years, I have seen doctors who only made me lose heart. All they ever told me was: **"Your knee will continue to degenerate. The only treatment for that is knee replacement, but not now. Go home, wait till your knee is thoroughly worn, and come back for an artificial knee."** *I am scared and devastated. My knee is sick, and my mind is sick, too.*

Many patients have told me similar stories over the years, but I have not told them to wait for knee replacement. I have advised them to intervene proactively with the KHPO. Fortunately for them, many of them have heeded my recommendation, and consequently they have kept their knees and got quality back in their lives.

The ACRFP reverses the degenerative course - visual evidence

Here are X-rays of two of my patients who received the ACRFP under KHPO treatment:

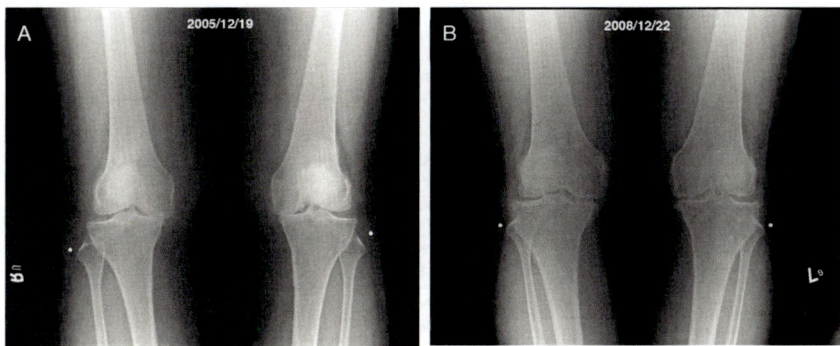

Fig. 3, the ACRFP has reversed the degenerative course: (A) A pre-operative view of a 58-year-old female patient having bilateral grade IV knee OA with subluxation (partial dislocation) of medial femoral condyle. Both knee received the ACRFP surgery. (B) Three years after the ACRFP, joint space has obviously opened up and the subluxation has improved.

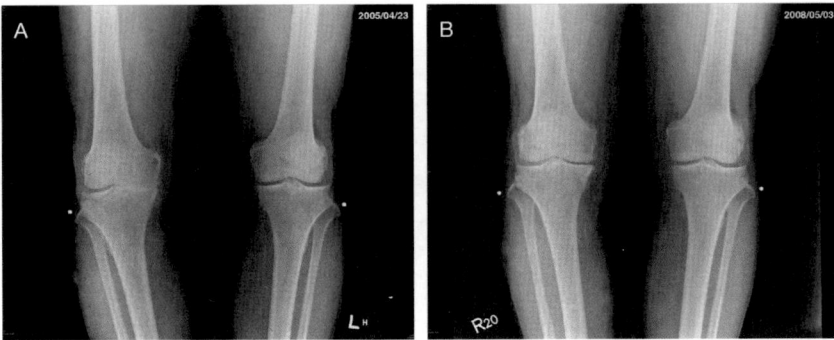

Fig. 4, the ACRFP has reversed the course of degeneration and deformity in a 70-year-old male patient. (A) The pre-operative view shows grade IV knee OA in his right knee, which was treated with the ACRFP. (B) Three years after the ACRFP, the joint space has reopened, and the femorotibial angle, a measurement of deformity, has improved from 7 degrees varus to 3 degrees varus. [Notice a narrower space between the legs in (B) than in (A)]

As these X-rays clearly show, the joint spaces of these patients have opened up after the ACRFP, and they are enjoying their new lives with little or no knee pain.

This book highlights what I have learned about and what my patients have benefited from the KHPO protocol.

The ACRFP is an effective alternative to knee replacement. Knee pain sufferers are advised to learn more about it and ask their doctors about it.

Shaw-Ruey Lyu, MD, PhD
Director, Joint Centre, Dalin Tzu Chi Hospital
Chiayi, Taiwan

Chapter 1 Terminology

Before I lay out how and why my "unconventional" treatment protocol for knee OA is effective, it is necessary to define a few terms that are used to describe the protocol. After you have perused these definitions, you may have already got a fairly good idea of what this protocol is about.

I have included some X-ray images in the book. When you read an X-ray of the knee, remember to flip sides: The leg on the left side of an X-ray is the right leg in real life (as if you were standing face-to-face).

1. Knee OA

    Osteoarthritis of the knee

2. Five major risk factors in the knee for knee OA according to our concept of KHPO

    (a) medial abrasion phenomenon

    (b) lateral compression phenomenon

    (c) synovitis

    (d) chondral flaps

    (e) meniscus tears

3. Conventional arthroscopic operations for knee OA

    Common conventional arthroscopic treatments for knee OA include arthroscopic lavage, debridement, chondroplasty, mosaicplasty, and resection of torn menisci. They are often considered ineffectual and over-utilised.

    These are **not** what this book is about.

4. The KHPO (Knee Health Promotion Option)

    The KHPO is the subject matter of this book.

Chapter 1

As the name indicates, the **KHPO is an alternative to conventional protocols for the treatment of knee OA**. Knee replacement is what conventional treatment protocols call for when the patient has exhausted all other available conventional treatments. **The KHPO offers the ACRFP as an additional option that is not available in the conventional protocols.**

KHPO is a multidisciplinary treatment protocol for OA knees that the author, *Dr. Shaw-Ruey Lyu*, has developed, evolved, and progressed. The protocol has been in use at his hospital since 2007. **It has so far saved thousands of patients from knee replacements while relieving their knee OA pains and restoring their knee function.**

A key idea in the KHPO protocol is to perform timely, proactive ACRFP procedures to remove all existing risk factors for knee OA from the knee cavity so it becomes hospitable for cartilage to function and regenerate.

This KHPO idea of early and proactive intervention to remove the risk factors for knee OA flies in the face of the conventional treatment protocols. A brief comparison follows. More detailed comparisons are provided in **Chapter 6**.

The conventional protocols are published by major medical academies to guide healthcare providers on how to treat their patients. These protocols basically call for pain management, physical therapy, and other conservative measures—without doing anything to eradicate the cause of knee OA. Often, knee replacement later becomes the only choice for patients.

In contrast, the KHPO eradicates the cause of knee OA early and proactively. Often, knee replacement becomes unnecessary.

5. ACRFP (arthroscopic cartilage regeneration facilitating procedure)

Chapter 1

The ACRFP is an umbrella procedure name for five member arthroscopic procedures. The goal of the ACRFP is to remove all existing risk factors for knee OA from the knee cavity so it becomes hospitable for cartilage to operate and regenerate.

The five member arthroscopic procedures are: AMR (arthroscopic medial release), PLR (percutaneous lateral release), synovectomy, chondroplasty, and partial meniscectomy, each of which removes a specific risk factor for knee OA according to our concept of KHPO.

The AMR is always performed during an ACRFP operation, but each of the other four member procedures is performed only when the corresponding risk factor is present. Therefore, an ACRFP session may include as few as one procedure (AMR) and as many as all five member procedures. This understanding sheds light on how the ACRFP is different from and indeed superior to the conventional arthroscopic treatments for knee OA.

6. AMR (arthroscopic medial release)

This procedure addresses this risk factor for knee OA: medial abrasion phenomenon.

(a) Removes hypertrophied medial plica. The AMR removes the abrasion phenomenon between the tight, fibrotic and hypertrophied medial plica and the opposite medial femoral condyle (the round bump on the femur where it articulates with the patella and tibia).

(b) Removes inflamed and thickened medial synovium and capsule.

(c) Adjusts and fine tunes the tension between patella and femoral condyle so the tension is appropriate for cartilage regeneration. The skill and experience of the surgeon are essential to delivering the required adjustment during the AMR operation.

Chapter 1

AMR is a novel procedure that the author devised to manage the **medial abrasion phenomenon**, a risk factor for knee OA. AMR is the core procedure of the ACRFP.

7. MAP (medial abrasion phenomenon)

Medial abrasion phenomenon is a common but little recognised phenomenon in OA knee patients caused by the repeated impingement between mediopatellar plica (medial plica) and the opposite medial femoral condyle during knee motion.

This phenomenon, according to the author's research team, is an important but almost always ignored cause of knee OA. Therefore, to cure knee OA, this phenomenon must be managed, hence the vital significance of the AMR procedure. This is why the AMR is the core procedure of the ACRFP.

8. MAS (medial abrasion syndrome)

Medial abrasion syndrome, named by the author, is a set of clinical symptoms and signs caused by medial abrasion phenomenon.

This syndrome can account for most of the symptoms that patients of knee OA may experience.

9. Medial plica (mediopatellar plica)

Medial plica is a fold of synovium. It normally does not cause problems, but a hypertrophied medial plica may cause the MAS as a result of repeated impingement between medial plica and the opposite medial femoral condyle during knee motion.

10. PCRFM (post-operative cartilage regeneration facilitating modalities)

Medial abrasion phenomenon, lateral compression phenomenon, synovitis, chondral debris, and torn menisci have been proven as the main causes of cartilage damage. After the ACRFP has removed these detrimental factors, the patient should engage in post-operative care of daily rehabilitation exercises for at least one year, and preferably for life.

Three exercises are respectively for quadriceps strengthening and soft tissue stretching (see Appendix II).

During the first 3 months after the ACRFP, the main objective of the rehabilitation is to prevent scar contracture, which may lead to the recurrence of medial abrasion phenomenon. Gentle, deep-bending and extending stretching exercises are encouraged after each session of a quadriceps strengthening exercise.

To facilitate cartilage regeneration, strict rules about engaging in appropriate daily activities and exercises should be followed during the first post-operative year (see Appendix III). The rationale for this precaution is to avoid repeated bending of the knee that might produce shearing forces harmful to cartilage regeneration. Prescribed muscle strengthening and soft tissue stretching exercises around the knee should be done as long as possible.

PCRFM—daily rehab exercise by the patient—is an integral part of a successful KHPO treatment. **Once the surgeon has done the ACRFP, the rest is, rightfully, in the hand of the patient.**

11. PLR (percutaneous lateral release)

    This procedure addresses this risk factor for knee OA: lateral compression phenomenon.

    PLR adjusts and fine tunes the tension between patella and femoral condyle so the tension is appropriate for cartilage regeneration.

12. Synovectomy

    This procedure addresses this risk factor for knee OA: synovitis.

    Synovectomy removes focal or generalised synovitis, which is harmful to the cartilage

13. Chondroplasty

    This procedure addresses this risk factor for knee OA: chondral flaps (torn cartilage).

    Chondroplasty removes chondral flaps, which will cause abnormal impingement or abrasion to the cartilage and cause damage.

14. Partial meniscectomy

    This procedure addresses this risk factor for knee OA: meniscus tears.

    Partial meniscectomy removes meniscus tears, which will cause abnormal impingement or abrasion to the cartilage and cause damage.

15. TKR or TKA

    Total Knee Replacement, Total Knee Arthroplasty

16. UKA or Uni-K

    Unicompartmental Knee Arthroplasty, Unicompartmental Knee Replacement, Partial Knee Replacement

Chapter 2 The KHPO in A Nutshell

In every phenomenon the beginning remains always the most notable moment.

- Thomas Carlyle, 1795-1881

Your knee hurts when you walk, sometimes even when you rest. You wish you wouldn't hurt so much, you wish your doctor knew what caused your knee pain, and, above all, you wish your doctor knew a better solution for you than knee replacement.

Our practice has identified a common but little recognised cause of knee osteoarthritis (knee OA), and in 2004 we devised an arthroscopic treatment option called arthroscopic cartilage regeneration facilitating procedure (ACRFP) that has (1) relieved thousands of patients of their knee pain without using analgesics, (2) helped open up the joint space in their knees, and (3) improved their mobility. The ACRFP has debunked the myth that cartilage in the knee naturally degenerates and proved that "degenerative arthritis of the knee" is a misnomer. A better name of the disease is "osteoarthritis of the knee".

Since 2007, our practice has further expanded the ACRFP into a comprehensive, multidisciplinary management protocol—the knee health promotion option (KHPO)—to treat patients with knee OA. The result shows the effectiveness of the KHPO in treating knee OA. Let's look at some facts.

Chapter 2

Most knee OA patients satisfied with their natural knees three years after their ACRFP, an arthroscopic surgery

> Between April 2010 and March 2011, I performed ACRFP under KHPO protocol on 536 knees of 317 patients to treat their knee OA. We followed up with them regularly, including X-rays, and we found that
>
> **94% of the patients with stage II knee OA,**
>
> **87.5% of the patients with stage III knee OA, and**
>
> **79.7% of the patients with stage IV knee OA**
>
> remained satisfied with their own knees three years after their ACRFP.

A few observations:

1. All of these patients, even those with stage IV knee OA, still keep their knees three years after the ACRFP. **Many of these patients have recovered well following the KHPO treatment, they have less or no knee pain, and they still walk around with their own knees.**

2. The sooner the ACRFP is performed, the better satisfied the patients have become.

3. These patients typically have not needed pain medicine for their knee OA soon after their ACRFP surgery.

Chapter 2

A Disease Process for Knee OA

So Nature deals with us, and takes away
Our playthings one by one, and by the hand
Leads us to rest so gently ...

- Henry Wadsworth Longfellow, 1807-1882

The conventional, mainstream medicine for knee OA has for a long time regarded it as the result of a natural degenerative process. They even classify it as a degenerative disease. Our research and clinical practice have found that characterisation to be misguided.

The following disease process for knee OA is based on our research that has spanned 15 years. We have published 12 scientific papers on this research. (See **Chapter 11**) The KHPO has been built on our knowledge about this disease process. Knowing how knee OA originates, evolves, and deteriorates has given us a solid foundation upon which to design and improve a focused treatment protocol that has field-proven to halt that deterioration process.

Here is the disease process that has so far still eluded the traditional mainstream medicine for knee OA.

Chapter 2

Medial Plica - the cause of medial abrasion phenomenon

You take a step, and this thing rubs on its neighbour once. You take another step, and it rubs on the neighbour another time. Without fail, the rubbing occurs with each step that you take, be it forward, upward, or downward. That rubbing may have painful consequences.

This thing that I am talking about is a small fold, a medial plica in anatomical lingo, in your knee (see Fig. 5). This fold is always touching its neighbour, the cartilage on the round bump on the lower inside end of your thighbone, also called medial femoral condyle. Each time you flex or extend your knee, the motion makes the fold rub on the opposite cartilage on the medial femoral condyle. This rubbing is usually not a problem if your medial plica is soft and small, or if you are a couch potato.

But if your plica becomes thick, or fibrous, or if you bend your knees a lot, then the rubbing may cause abrasion damage to both the fold and the cartilage opposite. Suppose you bend your knee just three thousand times a day (probably on the lower end of the activity spectrum), each of your knees bends a million times in a year. A fibrous medial plica rubbing the cartilage on the thigh bone a million times a year, year after year, may wear off the cartilage.

This rubbing is an important cause of knee OA.

Chapter 2

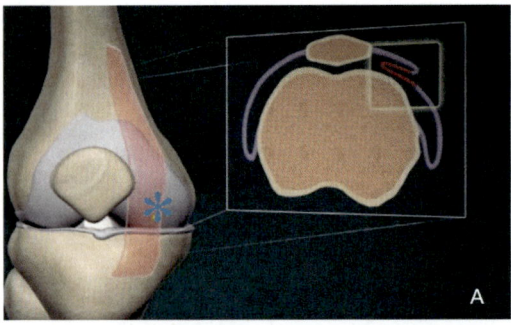
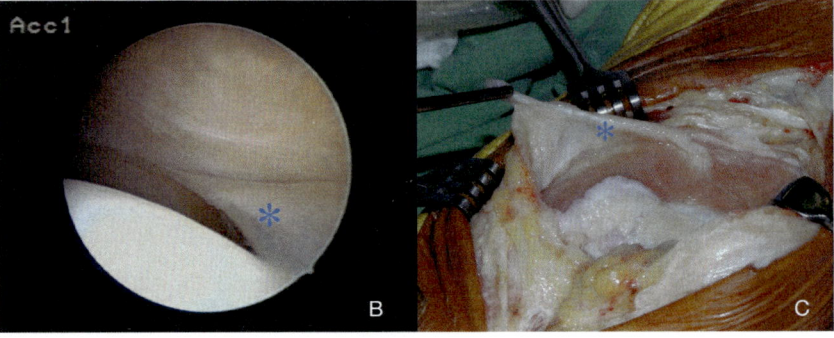

Fig. 5, medial plica (marked by *) is a fold of synovium (A); in young age, it is thin and soft as seen by arthroscopy (B); it will become thick and fibrotic in middle and old age as shown in the knee of this patient received total knee replacement (C).

Chapter 2

This kind of persistent, repetitive rubbing may cause

1. Abrasion damage to the chondrocyte and matrix of the medial femoral condyle
2. Synovitis around the plica, which leads to the excess production of cartilage degrading proteins and enzymes, such as IL-1β and MMP-3, to erode the cartilage
3. The debris and particles from the abrasion or erosions to settle at the bottom of the medial (inside, towards the centre) compartment of the knee. Gravity and particle size keep the debris near the bottom of that compartment, and the debris moves with knee movements, causing additional abrasion to weight-bearing areas of the knee. The particle size prevents the debris from passing freely to the lateral (outside, away from the centre) compartment of the knee, so the debris stays in, does damage to, and cause pain largely only in the medial compartment.

All this leaves the medial compartment filled with cartilage-damaging proteins, making it conducive to the self-destruction (apoptosis) of cartilage. This hostile environment comes about because of the medial abrasion phenomenon, not necessarily because of ageing.

Therefore, **"degenerative arthritis of the knee" is a misnomer.** The correct name of the disease is **"osteoarthritis of the knee"**.

Chapter 2

Medial abrasion phenomenon: an etiologic factor that inflicts three-pronged causative damage on an OA knee

Medial abrasion phenomenon is an etiologic factor for knee OA as illustrated in Figure 6. The repeated abrasion (easily a million times per year) between medial plica (the yellow curved line shown in Fig. 6) and the medial femoral condyle could inflict three-pronged damage on an OA knee.

Chapter 2

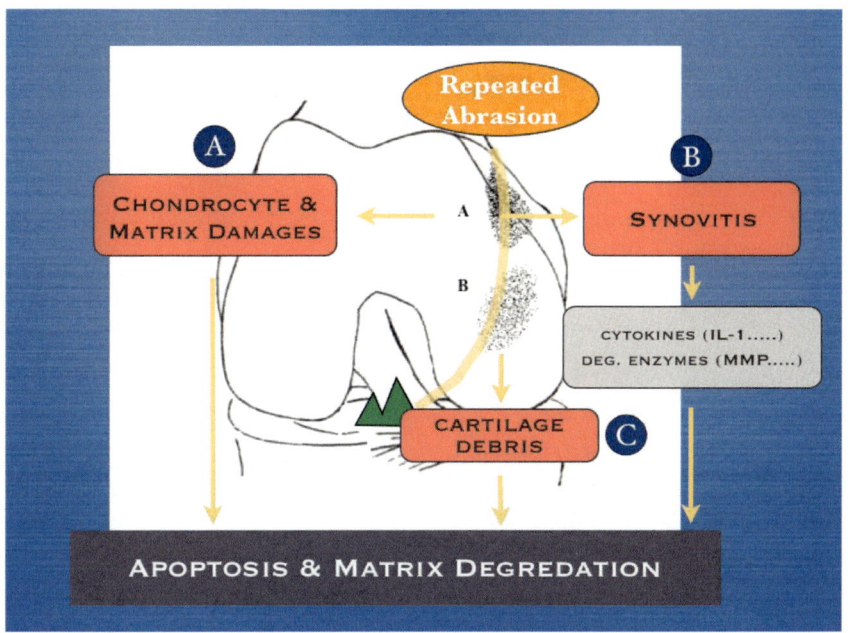

Fig. 6, medial abrasion phenomenon would cause: (A) chondrocyte and matrix damage from the direct mechanical shearing force (**physical abrasion**), (B) synovitis around medial plica that will produce cytokines, such as IL-1β, and cartilage-degrading enzymes, such as MMP-3, (**chemical erosion**), and (C) the debris and particles shedding down from the damaged cartilage will accumulate in the medial compartment, further causing **third-party abrasion** in weight bearing areas in the knee.

Depending on the size and severity of fibrosis of the medial plica, the abrasion itself will produce abnormal shearing force on the opposite cartilage of the medial femoral condyle and cause various degrees of cartilaginous damage. On the opposite side, this abrasion phenomenon causes repeated injury to the medial plica itself and results in focal synovitis that will trigger the production of cytokines such as IL-1β and then raise the production of cartilage-degrading enzymes such as MMP-3. The continuous shedding of cartilaginous debris and the production of cartilage-degrading enzymes make the whole medial compartment persistently in a condition that is detrimental to normal cartilage metabolism. Consequently, the so-called progressive degeneration ensues. Moreover, the painful sensation of inflammation of medial plica might evoke a reflex contracture of the pes anserinus muscle group and increase the loading of the medial compartment, thus further jeopardising the cartilage.

According to our theory, the medial abrasion phenomenon, if present, may persistently contribute to an environment in the knee that (a) is inhospitable to the cartilage in the medial compartment of the involved knee, (b) disturbs normal cartilage metabolism, and (c) thus brings about a disease process that many people mistakenly call "degeneration".

Degeneration is a result, not a cause, of knee OA. One important but neglected cause of knee OA, **according to our research**, is the medial abrasion phenomenon.

Chapter 2

Simple can be harder than complex.

You have to work hard to get your thinking clean to make it simple.

- Steve Jobs, 1955-2011

We have pinpointed a cause of knee OA, so now we can look at how to treat it.

An intervention process—the KHPO, a treatment protocol for knee OA

All physicians strive to use non-surgical therapies to relieve pain for their patients with knee OA. But when such measures fail, surgeons typically have one last resort, which is knee replacement, because they have nothing else in their repertoire.

Like them, we also do knee replacement in our practice, but only as a last resort. Often we do not need to resort to knee replacement because, unlike them, we do have at our disposal a potent alternative treatment. We call that treatment the KHPO, or Knee Health Promotion Option.

Based on the knowledge in the disease process, we have designed the KHPO to first conservatively treat knee OA to manage the symptoms. If that works, great, but if that fails, we proceed to arthroscopic surgery to eradicate a root cause of knee OA, and the result, as shown above, has been quite remarkable.

Chapter 2

The KHPO protocol

Here is how we do it in our practice (Fig. 7).

1. Based on the extent of joint space narrowing, the presence of osteophytes, the femorotibial angle, and the stability of the joint, we assign each patient to a clinical stage of severity for OA knee, ranging from I to V, with stage V being the most severe.
2. As shown in Table 1, most of stage II, all of stage III, and some of stage IV patients are advised to receive the ACRFP. The rest of stage IV patients and all of stage V patients are advised to receive arthroplasty (unicompartmental or total knee replacement).
3. Before the ACRFP surgery, all except stage V patients are advised to undergo a conservative treatment for at least three months that is supervised by a case manager or a nurse on our staff. The patients get to know the disease process, they learn that the medial abrasion phenomenon is an important etiologic factor for their knee pain, and they are urged to commit to the KHPO treatment protocol, which requires the patients to (1) modify their daily activities and exercises to avoid repeatedly bending their knees (see Appendix III) and (2) perform three rehabilitation exercises every day (see Appendix II).

   If the conservative treatment alleviates a patient's knee pain, he or she stays on that treatment. Only when the conservative treatment has failed will the patient actually receive the ACRFP surgery.
4. The ACRFP surgery is followed by at least 12 months of post-operative cartilage regeneration facilitating modalities (PCRFM), the purpose of which is to rekindle the natural repair process to rehabilitate damaged cartilage in the knees. Usually, we prescribe pain medications only for the few days immediately following surgery, but nothing afterwards because they do not need them.

   During the first three months after the ACRFP surgery, the prescribed rehabilitation exercises are primarily to prevent surgical scars from hardening. Such contracture may lead medial abrasion phenomenon to recur.

Chapter 2

5. To avoid exerting shearing force harmful to cartilage regeneration, a recuperating patient should **avoid repeatedly bending their knees more than 50 degrees**. Therefore, sufferers of OA knees may engage in activities such as walking, jogging, golfing, and swimming freestyle or butterfly strokes. But they are advised to refrain from knee-damaging activities such as climbing up or down stairs, mountain climbing, squatting (such as gardening), bicycling, and swimming breaststroke (see Appendix III).

6. One year after surgery, if the knee OA improves, the patient simply continues doing the prescribed daily rehabilitation exercises and no other action is necessary. They may resume their normal daily activities and exercise. Things look good.

If the knee OA fails to improve or gets worse, the patient is advised to receive total or partial knee replacement.

Chapter 2

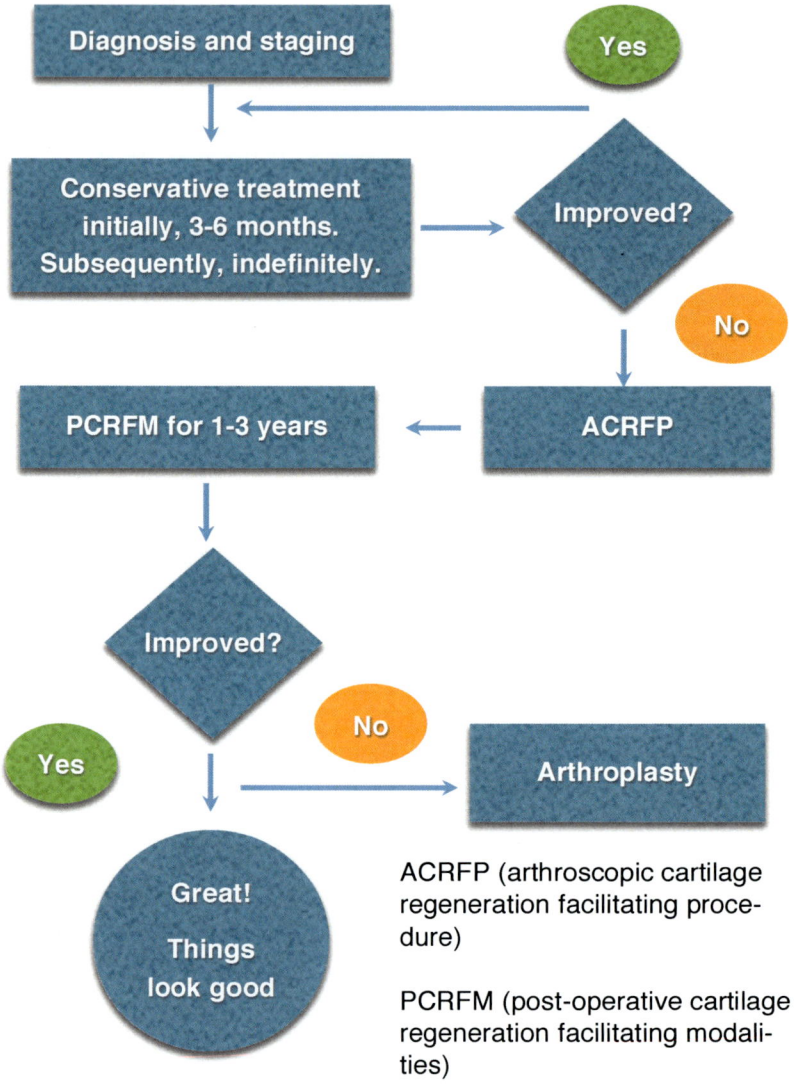

Fig. 7, knee health promotion option (KHPO) flow chart for knee OA treatment

Table 1.

Recommendation of treatment option for different stage of knee OA

Stage	ACRFP	Uni-K	TKA
I	-	-	-
II	++	-	-
III	+++	-	-
IV	+	+++	++
V	-	++	+++

ACRFP = Arthroscopic Cartilage Regeneration Facilitating Procedure
Uni-K = Unicompartmental Knee Arthroplasty
TKA = Total Knee Arthroplasty

Chapter 2

Types of surgical procedures in KHPO if conservative treatment fails

There are two types of surgical procedures in the KHPO protocol: arthroscopic surgery and open surgery.

1. The arthroscopic surgery is called ACRFP (arthroscopic cartilage regeneration facilitating procedure), which is the umbrella name for a set of arthroscopic procedures that is to, in one fell swoop, eradicate the five main known risk factors for knee OA according to our concept of treatment, namely, medial abrasion phenomenon, lateral compression phenomenon, synovitis, chondral flaps, and torn menisci.

The arthroscopic surgery to treat these risk factors are arthroscopic medial release (AMR), percutaneous lateral release (PLR), synovectomy, chondroplasty, and partial meniscectomy, respectively.

The AMR is a novel procedure that our practice has invented, evolved, and matured to relieve knee pain and restore knee function. So far, thousands of patients of knee OA have benefited.

The AMR includes (1) the removal of hypertrophied medial plica, (2) the removal of inflamed and thickened medial synovium and capsule, and (3) the adjustment to the tension between patella and femoral condyle so the tension is conducive to cartilage regeneration.

The ACRFP always includes the AMR as its anchor procedure. If another risk factor is also present, then the appropriate procedure is added to the ACRFP cocktail. For example, the presence of synovitis adds synovectomy to the ACRFP lineup. Therefore, the ACRFP may contain as few as one procedure (the AMR) and as many as five procedures. The exact makeup of an ACRFP is dictated by the risk factors that are

Chapter 2

actually present in a patient's knee. We tailor each ACRFP to meet a patient's unique needs.

In short, the ACRFP, in one go, eliminates existing detrimental factors in the knee to **make the knee a more hospitable place for damaged cartilage to stop degenerating and start regenerating.**

After the ACRFP, a root cause of knee OA—the rubbing between medial plica and the facing medial femoral condyle that gives rise to the medial abrasion syndrome (MAS)—will not appear again. The reason is simple: the medial plica is no longer there; the ACRFP has cut it off. If it is not there, it cannot rub and cause damage.

2. Open surgery: This refers to partial or total knee replacement operations (PKR or TKR). Such operations are utilised in the KHPO protocol only as a last resort, in the event that the ACRFP has failed.

Chapter 2

Two reminders:

1. The KHPO protocol, though consisting mainly of arthroscopic surgery, does include knee replacement (TKR or UKR), but only as a last resort when the arthroscopic operation (ACRFP) has failed to relieve knee pain.

2. The knee replacement surgeries in our practice include one extra step that is not normally done by other surgeons: the eradication of the medial abrasion phenomenon. About 30 percent of patients who receive *traditional* arthroplasty—with the pathologic medial plica intact in the knee—continue to suffer knee pain in spite of the new prostheses that are advertised to end their knee pain once and for all. In contrast, that percentage for *KHPO* arthroplasty—with pathologic medial plica excised—recipients in our practice is 0 %. A pathologic medial plica could cause problems—even with prostheses in place—so it is important to remove it during the surgery to treat knee OA, whether it be the ACRFP or a knee replacement

Chapter 3 What Has ACRFP Done for Patients? It Has Helped Their Cartilage Regrow

The ACRFP removes all present risk factors for knee OA from an inflicted knee, so the knee becomes more hospitable to cartilage to regenerate. Revitalised cartilage not only relieves clinical symptoms but also reverses the course of degeneration.

Many in academia have claimed that cartilage does not regenerate, perhaps because they have been unable to prove that it does. However, in our practice, we have repeatedly seen cartilage regrow in our patients after they have received the ACRFP. And I am talking not about just a few lucky patients but about most of them that number in the thousands.

They have told us that they have experienced pain relief in their knees and they have been able to resume their normal activities.

We have arthroscopic and X-ray images to prove our claim. A picture is worth a thousand words, and I will show a few of them here.

Chapter 3

The ACRFP reverses cartilage degeneration:
Visual evidence 1

Case 1: Worn Cartilage Regrows (3 years)

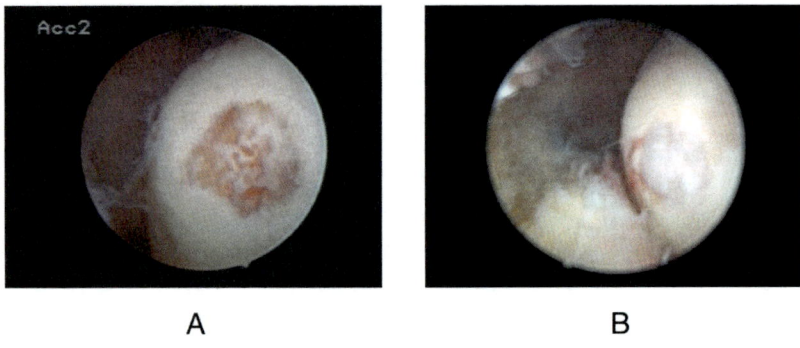

A   B

Fig. 8, cartilage regeneration demonstrated in the medial compartment of the left knee of a 56-year-old female who had stage III knee OA: (A) Her cartilage had eroded and thinned (pink area) on the medial femoral condyle opposite her pathologic medial plica, which the ACRFP removed. (B) The thinned cartilage has grown back (white has covered the pink) three year later, when this image was taken during a second-look arthroscopy of the same knee. Image (B) clearly shows that cartilage regenerates in a hospitable knee cavity, which the ACRFP has provided. Second-look arthroscopy is generally not necessary for ACRFP patients because follow-up X-rays are usually sufficient to show the progress of their knee. However, this female patient needed the second arthroscopy because her ACRFP-treated knee suffered from hemoarthrosis after she had fallen down in an accident.

Chapter 3

The ACRFP reverses cartilage degeneration:

Visual evidence 2

Case 2: The ACRFP Reverses the Degenerative Course (1 year)

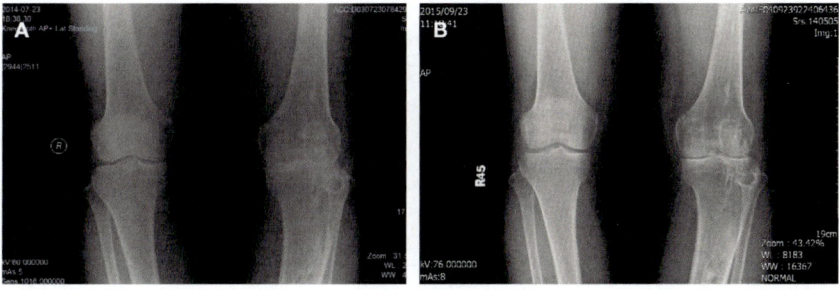

Fig. 9, the ACRFP has reversed the degenerative course:
(A) A pre-operative view of a 53-year-old male patient having grade III OA in his right knee and grade IV OA in his left knee. Both knee received the ACRFP surgery. (B) One year after the ACRFP, joint spaces have obviously opened up.

Chapter 3

The ACRFP reverses cartilage degeneration:

Visual evidence 3

Case 3: The ACRFP Reverses the Degenerative Course (2 years)

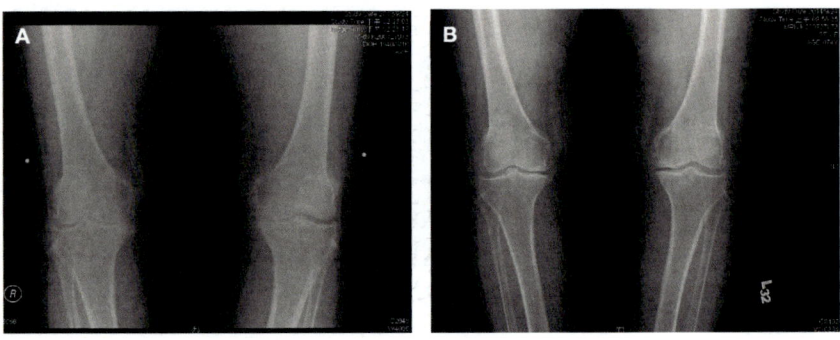

Fig. 10, the ACRFP has reversed the degenerative course:
(A) A pre-operative view of a 63-year-old female patient having bilateral grade IV knee OA. Both knees received the ACRFP surgery. (B) Two years after the ACRFP, joint spaces have obviously opened up.

Chapter 3

The ACRFP reverses cartilage degeneration:

Visual evidence 4

Case 4: The ACRFP Reverses the Degenerative Course (3 years)

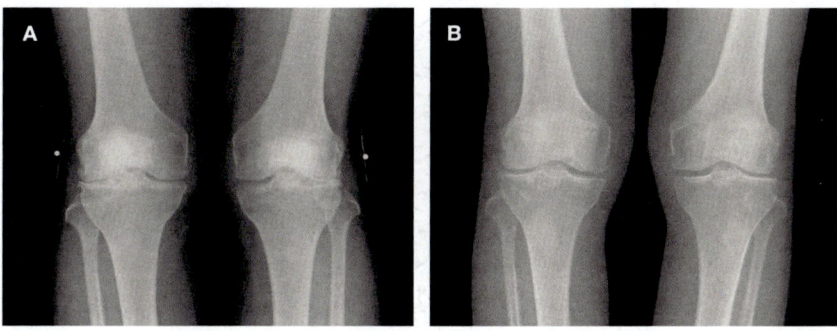

Fig. 11, the ACRFP has reversed the course of degeneration and deformity in a 70-year-old female patient: (A) The pre-operative view shows bilateral grade IV knee OA, which was treated with the ACRFP. (B) Three years after the ACRFP, the joint spaces have reopened.

Chapter 3

The ACRFP reverses cartilage degeneration:

Visual evidence 5

Case 5: The ACRFP Reverses the Degenerative Course (8 years)

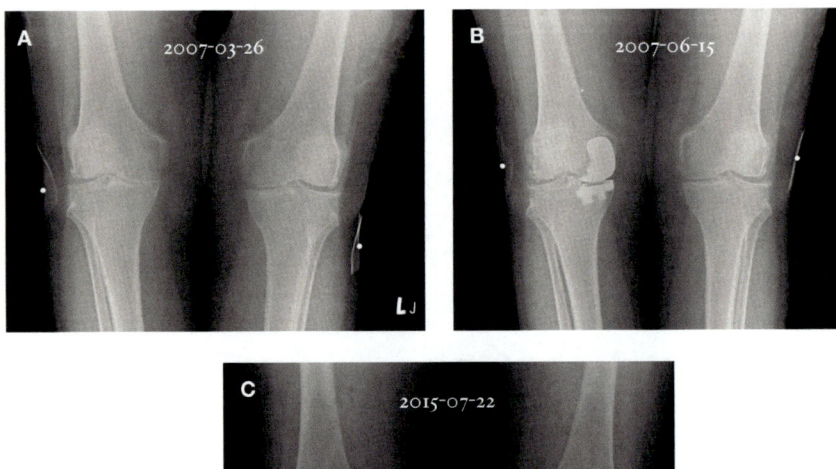

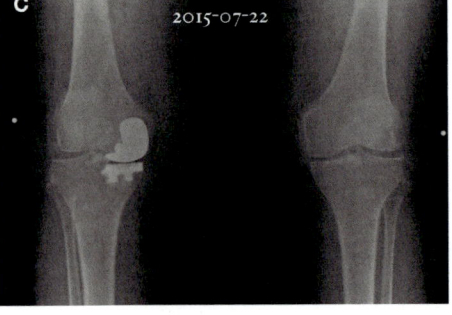

Fig. 12, the ACRFP has reversed the degenerative course:
(A) A pre-operative view of a 65-year-old female patient having grade IV OA in her right knee and grade III OA in her left knee. (B) Unicompartmental arthroplasty was performed for her right knee and ACRFP was performed for her left knee. (C) **Eight years later**, joint space has obviously opened up over her left knee (that was treated with the ACRFP).

Chapter 3

The ACRFP reverses cartilage degeneration:

Visual evidence 6

Case 6: The ACRFP Reverses Cartilage Degeneration (self-control)

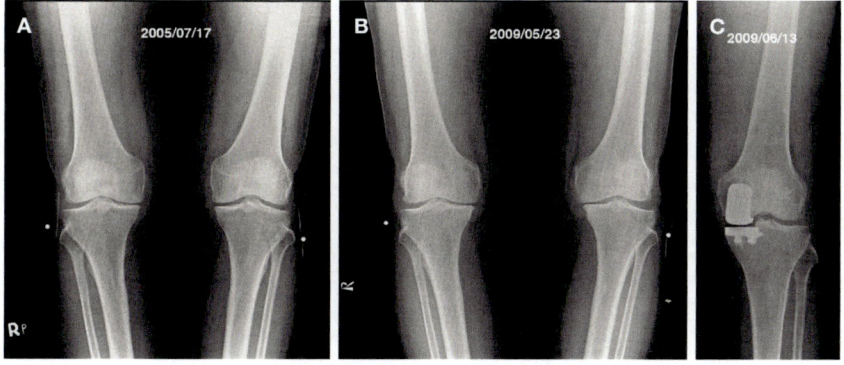

Fig. 13, (A) This is an example of self-control from a 61-year-old male with grade III knee OA over medial compartment of the right knee and grade II OA over medial compartment of the left knee. The right knee (left in X-ray) received the ACRFP but the left knee did not. (B) 46 months later, he came back for a treatment of the marked disability in his left knee — which did not receive the ACRFP. His right knee, by contrast, was in excellent condition. The degeneration process has ceased on his ACRFP-treated right knee but has continued on his untreated left knee that has led to severe deformity. [Notice a wider space between the legs in (B) than in (A)]. (C) Consequently, his left knee received unicompartmental arthroplasty (partial knee replacement).

Chapter 3

The ACRFP reverses cartilage degeneration:

Visual evidence 7

Case 7: The ACRFP Reverses the Degenerative Course (2 years)

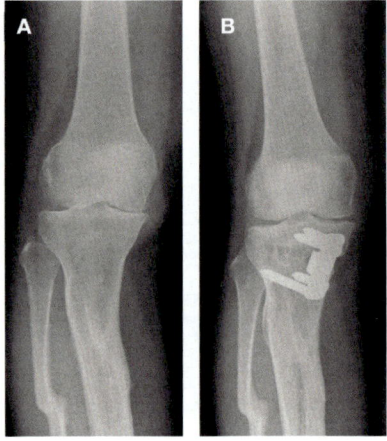

Fig. 14, an example of the ACRFP and high tibia osteotomy (the procedure to correct the deformity of a bone) working together to widen the joint space in the knee of a 58-year-old female with grade IV OA in her right knee. (A) is before the ACRFP surgery and (B) is two years after the surgery. Significant improvements can be seen in (B).

Chapter 4 The Hidden Hazards of Ineffective Conservative Treatments

In short, the main hazards are patient suffering, delayed treatments, unchecked knee deterioration, and lost opportunities to keep your knees, in order of increasing clinical significance.

Treating a disease without knowing its cause is like waging a war without knowing who and where the enemy is. It does not take a Sun Tzu to know that nobody can win that kind of a clueless war. Unfortunately, that is exactly how the current medical establishment is fighting the war on knee OA. No wonder its member doctors are losing the war quite badly, often forcing them to resort to knee replacement.

Therefore, it matters a great deal to choose doctors who know about the risk factors for knee OA. The treatments that they recommend are more likely to be effective.

Many physicians put their patients of knee OA on conventional conservative treatments first. That is prudent. However, many such treatments are not effective. **The following conventional conservative treatments are usually NOT effective: painkillers, glucosamine, chondroitin, and intra-articular injections such as hyaluronic acid and PRP (platelet-rich plasma).**

The following will show why you should be alerted if you are getting only such ineffective conservative treatments for your knee OA.

A treatment that does not remove the underlying cause of knee OA is unlikely to be effective. Furthermore, your knee continues to deteriorate while you undergo the ineffective treatment. The deterioration may even acceler-

Chapter 4

ate because your pains are dulled and masked by such treatment, so you may overuse without constrain and harm the jeopardised knee.

Pain is a protective mechanism. Tampering with pain mechanisms and temporarily blocking pain without treating the underlying cause of knee OA, which many conservative treatments tend to do, exposes the patient to hidden risks. Pains or no pains, the underlying causes, unless removed, continue to undermine the knee inexorably, and the disease continues to worsen. Patients who undergo conventional treatments run the risk of wasting away the best time for effective interventions. The best window for treatment, once gone, may never return. The disease waits for no one.

Chapter 4

Ineffective treatments cost you much more than money

> **No amount of money can buy back the months or years that you have wasted on ineffective treatments.**
>
> Those are critical time, during which your knees continue to deteriorate, and during which effective treatments such as the ACRFP, may still save you from knee replacement:
>
> If your physician keeps avoiding effective treatments, thus allowing your knee to continue deteriorating for too long, it is possible that even those effective treatments cannot help you keep your knee.
>
> **You deserve better care than those ineffective treatments. You deserve to keep your knees. You are advised to evaluate your treatment and decline ineffective treatments.**

Chapter 4

How may a patient gauge the effectiveness of a proposed treatment?

Ask your knee doctor

- To describe what may have caused your knee OA (and don't take "degenerative" or "ageing" for an answer) and

- Whether or not his or her proposed treatment removes that cause.

A treatment that does not eradicate the cause of knee OA is troubling because

- It's not effective.

- It wastes valuable time during which your OA knees continue to deteriorate, maybe to the point that even the ACRFP cannot help. You may waste time and miss out on the service and benefit of a viable treatment such as the KHPO.

- The knee degenerates even faster since the protective mechanism of pain is temporally blocked by these treatments and you continue to use or overuse the jeopardised knee as usual, exacerbating the disease.

Chapter 4

Everything that you do is a step in one direction or another.

- Henry van Dyke, 1852-1933

You need to be certain that your treatment is taking you in the direction of health rather than more sufferings.

There are a myriad of conservative treatments, all claiming effectiveness against knee OA. My sincere advice to you is:

Let the patients beware!

Let me just show a few popular conservative treatments below. See for yourself how they have caused unfortunate, truly unnecessary, and sometimes irreversible consequences. Just because a treatment is popular does not mean you should try it.

Chapter 4

Typical course by conservative treatments

The annual rate of progression in subjects diagnosed with knee OA has been reported as approximately 4% per year.

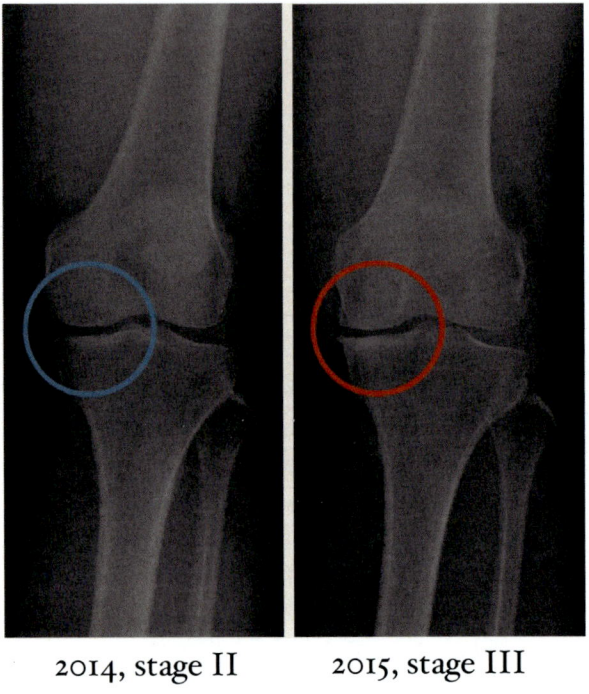

2014, stage II   2015, stage III

Fig. 15, this patient received conventional conservative treatment including painkillers, glucosamine, and intra-articular injections of hyaluronic acid and PRP (platelet-rich plasma). Her knee deteriorated (from stage II to III) within one year's time.

Chapter 4

Do painkillers halt cartilage attrition?

The answer is a resounding **"No!"**

Treatments that do not eradicate the cause of knee OA will not stop cartilage from wearing off. Conventional conservative treatments, including painkillers, are such treatments. Here is a proof.

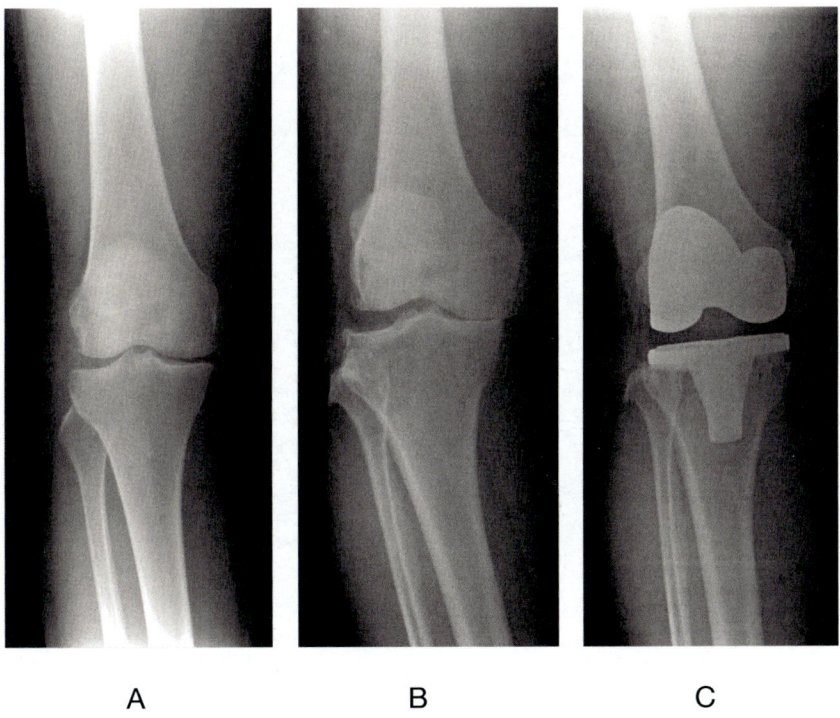

A   B   C

Fig. 16, the X-rays show a patient with stage III of knee OA (A), for whom a doctor elsewhere prescribed anti-inflammatory and analgesic drugs for two and a half years. By the end of that 30-month period, his knee has deteriorated to stage V, (B), which was followed by a total knee replacement, (C).

Chapter 4

Do steroids halt cartilage degeneration?

The answer is a resounding **"No!"**

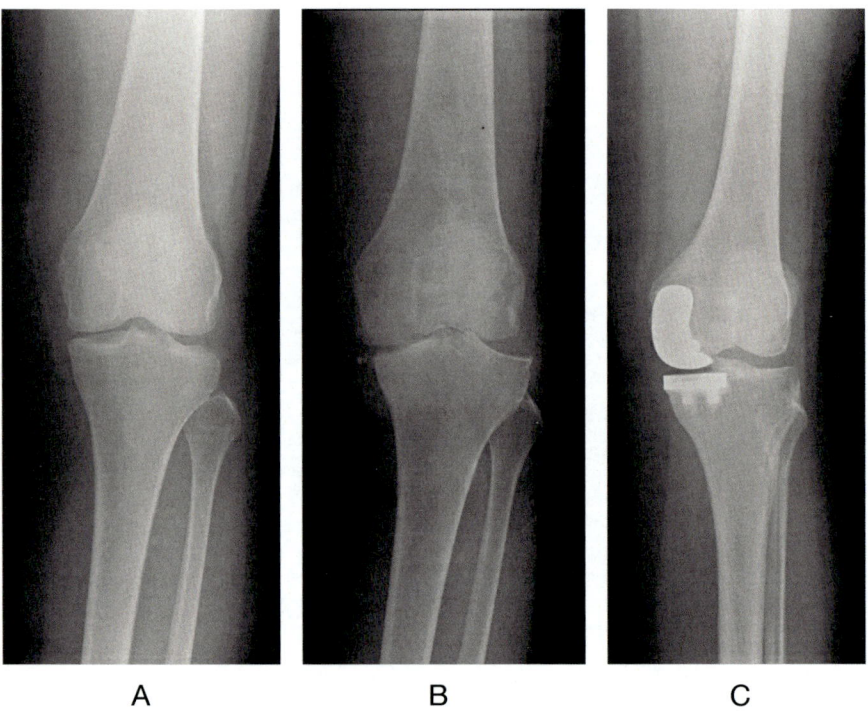

Fig. 17, (A) a stage III OA knee before taking steroids, (B) after taking steroids for 10 months during which the degeneration of the cartilage accelerated to the point of requiring a medial unicompartmental knee arthroplasty (partial knee replacement) (C).

Chapter 4

Are glucosamine and chondroitin effective against knee OA?

Glucosamine and chondroitin possess anti-inflammatory and analgesic properties, so they are capable of delivering relief to sufferers of knee OA rapidly, in just a few days. Be aware, though, that this is merely relief of symptoms. The underlying cause of knee OA remains untreated and intact, and it continues to cause damage.

Credible scientific studies have pointed out that taking glucosamine or chondroitin does not stop the deterioration of knee OA.

Chapter 4

Are hyaluronic acid (HA) injections effective against knee OA?

> If I may weigh in on this issue, I will offer what I have seen in my practice, not exactly scientific, but the opinions of large number of patients who have used the product.
>
> By the time patients come to my clinic, most of them have already tried other therapies or have been treated by other physicians. A vast majority of them, eight or nine out of ten, have told me that they have received hyaluronic acid injections elsewhere for their knee OA. Their opinions about hyaluronic acid injections are divided, about a half of them saying the injections have helped them and the other half rejecting that notion. **That makes hyaluronic acid injections about as effective as placebos**.
>
> Now I will offer what I have seen clinically. I have observed sequelae of HA injections in hundreds of these patients:
> 1. Severe fibrosis of synovium membrane, joint capsule, or fat pad as a result of reaction to multiple HA injections or accidental extra-articular injections. I often needed to take extra time and effort to clean these up when I performed the ACRFP to eradicate the cause of knee OA.
> 2. Bacterial or fungal infections after multiple HA injections may totally destroy cartilage and necessitates complicated management including long term antibiotics and salvage arthroplasty.

Chapter 4

Are platelet-rich plasma (PRP) injections effective against knee OA?

> With high profile endorsements, PRP injections have gotten popular. There were dozens of clinical studies on PRP in recent years, but they all share some shortcomings: (1) a short follow-up period of just 6 to 12 months, (2) a lack of control groups, (3) based on patients' subjective descriptions, and (4) a lack of objective evidence such as X-rays or arthroscopic images.
>
> These studies conclude that
> 1. PRP injections are more effective for younger patients with earlier-stage knee OA.
> 2. Some studies indicate that PRP injections are more effective and longer lasting than hyaluronic acid (HA) injections while other studies find no difference between them.
> 3. The effectiveness of PRP injections diminishes with time.
> 4. Evidence does not support definitive conclusions on the effectiveness of PRP injections.
>
> **PRP injections remain an unproven and costly treatment for knee OA. There is insufficient evidence to support the long-term effectiveness of PRP injections for knee OA, and there is no objective evidence to show that PRP helps cartilage regenerate.**

Chapter 5 Why is the ACRFP Better for the Knees? Its Distinctions and Advantages

What is the ACRFP?

Based on our basic research about and clinical observations in medial abrasion phenomenon, we designed the **arthroscopic cartilage regeneration facilitating procedure (ACRFP)** as an integrated, comprehensive, and novel arthroscopic surgery that aims to remove all existing risk factors of knee OA from the knee, hence making the knee a more hospitable place for the cartilage inside to regenerate.

What are the benefits of the ACRFP?

Simply put, the ACRFP (1) eradicates the medial abrasion phenomenon and inflamed synovium and capsule, (2) decompresses the patello-femoral joint, (3) restores soft tissue balance around the patella, (4) removes other known risk factors (synovitis, meniscus tears and chondral flaps) of knee OA, and (5) consequently improves the environment in the knee so it is more hospitable to cartilage regeneration.

When reading my research papers about the KHPO protocol and its components, such as the ACRFP, physicians often hurry to mistakenly conclude that ACRFP is just another version of conventional arthroscopic procedure for knee OA.

Moreover, since we emphasise that medial abrasion phenomenon is an important cause of knee OA, and the phenomenon involves medial plica, ACRFP has always been confused with arthroscopic resection of medial plica—a very simple procedure.

Chapter 5

Because conventional arthroscopic procedures have been repeatedly proven to be an ineffective treatment for knee OA and arthroscopic resection of medial plica is a part, albeit a small part, of ACRFP, **they jump to the mistaken conclusion that ACRFP could not be effective and that ACRFP is just another sham operation for knee OA,** notwithstanding the fact that I have used the ACRFP to treat thousands patients of knee OA with remarkable success.

Their misunderstanding is unfortunate. Because of these surgeons' misunderstanding, their patients may have lost out and continue to lose out on the benefits of the KHPO, and, worse, patients may have lost their knees in the past and may continue to lose their knees in the future.

So I have included in this book testimonials from my patients (see **Chapter 9**) on behalf of the ACRFP.

And I will clearly point out the significant differences between the ACRFP under KHPO protocol and conventional arthroscopic procedures for knee OA. **These differences make the ACRFP superior to the conventional arthroscopic procedures for knee OA.**

Common conventional arthroscopic treatments for knee OA include arthroscopic lavage, debridement, chondroplasty, mosaicplasty, and arthroscopic resection of torn menisci. They are often considered ineffective and over-utilised.

The ACRFP, especially the AMR portion, should not be confused with any of these procedures. The ACRFP is different from all of them.

$$\text{ACRFP} \neq \text{but} > \text{arthroscopic debridement}$$
$$\text{ACRFP} \neq \text{but} > \text{medial plica resection}$$
$$\text{ACRFP} = \text{a technique- and experience-demanding procedure}$$

Chapter 5

Is ACRFP under KHPO better than the conventional arthroscopic procedures?

The ACRFP under KHPO is a comprehensive treatment protocol for knee OA. It has many integrated remedial treatment components that are deployed when necessary **to eradicate all the major risk factors for knee OA** that are present.

On the other hand, the *conventional arthroscopic procedures and arthroscopic resection of medial plica lack most of the required remedial actions*. Therefore, they are not effective treatments for knee OA, they should not be mistaken for the ACRFP under KHPO, and they cannot be expected to deliver the same efficacy as that which the ACRFP under KHPO has reliably delivered.

Chapter 5

Differences between ACRFP, conventional arthroscopic procedures for knee OA, and arthroscopic resection of medial plica

Let me point out major differences between (1) the ACRFP, (2) common conventional arthroscopic treatments for knee OA (arthroscopic lavage, debridement, chondroplasty, mosaicplasty, lateral release, synovectomy, partial meniscectomy), and (3) arthroscopic resection of medial plica.

Each of the ACRFP member procedures is performed to remove a specific risk factor for knee OA

Chapter 5

Risk factors for knee OA

> **The five primary risk factors for knee OA** are:
>
> 1. Meidal abrasion phenomenon
> 2. Lateral compression phenomenon
> 3. Synovitis
> 4. Chondral flaps
> 5. Meniscus tears
>
> The ACRFP removes all these risk factors.
>
> Each ACRFP member procedure is performed to remove a specific risk factor, if present, for knee OA.
>
> After the ACRFP surgery, **two additional risk factors** may emerge. They are the result of patients not following post-operative instructions.
>
> 6. Recurrence of scarring, or fibrosis
> 7. Patients deviate from their daily rehab exercises or lose contact with the program.

Chapter 5

Risk factor (1): medial abrasion phenomenon

The remedial actions needed include (a) removal of hypertrophied medial plica, (b) removal of inflamed and thickened medial synovium and capsule, and (c) adjusting and fine tuning the tension between patella and femoral condyle so the tension is appropriate for cartilage regeneration.

The ACRFP performs all three remedial actions by the Arthroscopic Medial Release (AMR) to: (a) excise the medial plica, (b) remove inflamed and thickened medial synovium and capsule, and (c) adjust and fine tune the tension between patella and femoral condyle. The skill and experience of the surgeon are essential to delivering the required adjustment during AMR operations.

Conventional arthroscopic procedures do sometimes remove hypertrophied medial plica. They do not remove inflamed and thickened medial synovium and capsule, nor do they make the required tension adjustments.

An arthroscopic resection of medial plica removes hypertrophied medial plica. It does not remove inflamed and thickened medial synovium and capsule, nor does it make the required tension adjustments.

Risk factor (2): lateral compression phenomenon

The remedial action needed includes adjusting and fine tuning the tension between patella and femoral condyle so the tension is appropriate for cartilage regeneration.

The ACRFP performs the remedial action through a member procedure: the percutaneous lateral release (PLR).

Conventional arthroscopic procedures sometimes perform this remedial action.

An arthroscopic resection of medial plica does not perform this remedial action.

Chapter 5

Risk factor (3): synovitis

The remedial action needed includes the removal of focal or generalised synovitis, which is harmful to the cartilage.

The ACRFP perform the remedial action through a member procedure: synovectomy.

Synovectomy is also a conventional arthroscopic procedure. The stand-alone conventional synovectomy does perform the remedial action.

An arthroscopic resection of medial plica sometimes performs this remedial action.

Risk factor (4): chondral flaps

The remedial action needed includes chondroplasty for the removal of chondral flaps, which will cause abnormal impingement of or abrasion on the cartilage and cause damage.

The ACRFP sometimes performs this remedial action.

Chondroplasty is also a conventional arthroscopic procedure. The stand-alone conventional chondroplasty does perform this remedial action.

An arthroscopic resection of medial plica does not perform this remedial action.

Risk factor (5): meniscus tears

The remedial action needed includes partial meniscectomy for the removal of meniscus tears, which will cause abnormal impingement of or abrasion on the cartilage and cause damage.

The ACRFP sometimes performs this remedial action.

Chapter 5

Partial meniscectomy is also a conventional arthroscopic procedure. The stand-alone conventional partial meniscectomy does perform this remedial action.

An arthroscopic resection of medial plica does not perform this remedial action.

Risk factor (6): recurrence of scarring or fibrosis

The remedial action needed includes the three daily rehabilitation exercises (see Appendix II).

The ACRFP emphasises this action. This is an at-home, life-long task that the patient must undertake every day to prevent post-operative scarring that may lead to severe fibrosis.

Conventional arthroscopic procedures do not emphasise this action. A resection without the accompanying rehab exercises makes scarring, hence the pain, worse.

An arthroscopic resection of medial plica does not emphasise this action. A resection without the accompanying rehab exercises makes scarring, hence the pain, worse.

Risk factor (7): patients deviate from their daily rehab exercises or lose contact with the program

The remedial action calls for a case manager to carefully monitor, follow up, supervise, and talk with patients on an on-going basis—offering a lot of handholding to keep patients on track.

The ACRFP under KHPO emphasises this action.

Conventional arthroscopic procedures do not emphasise this action.

An arthroscopic resection of medial plica does not emphasise this action.

Chapter 5

Summary of differences between ACRFP, conventional arthroscopic procedures for knee OA and simple arthroscopic resection of medial plica

RF	Remedial Action	ACRFP	CAP	ARMP
1a	Remove hypertrophied medial plica	Yes	Sometimes	Yes
1b	Remove inflamed and thickened medial synovium and capsule	Yes	No	No
1c	Adjust the tension between patella and femoral condyle	Yes	No	No
2	Adjust the tension between patella and femoral condyle	Yes	Sometimes	No
3	Remove focal or generalised synovitis	Yes	Sometimes	Sometimes
4	Remove chondral flaps	Sometimes	Sometimes	No
5	Remove meniscus tears	Sometimes	Sometimes	No
6	Daily rehabilitation exercises	Yes	Not emphasised	Not emphasised
7	Monitored by case managers	Yes	Not emphasised	Not emphasised

Table 2. This table summarises the differences between the ACRFP under the KHPO protocol (ACRFP), conventional arthroscopic procedures for knee OA (CAP), and the arthroscopic resection of medial plica (ARMP) for each risk factor (RF).

Chapter 5

Summary of KHPO procedures and what they treat

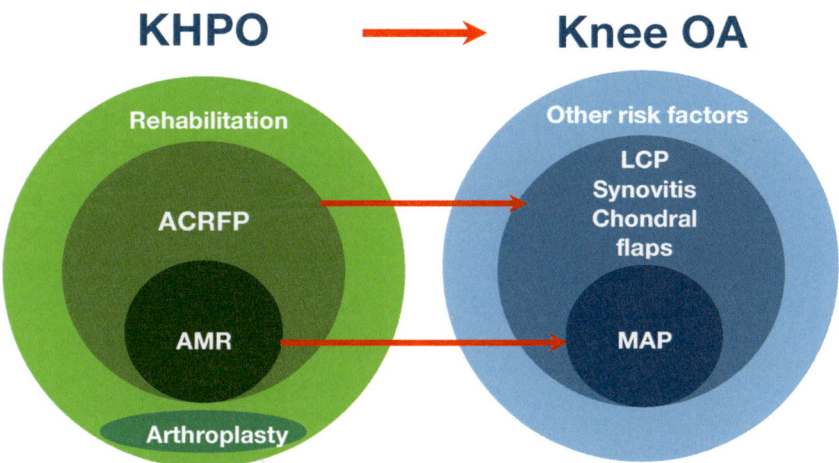

Fig. 18, summary of the strategy and surgical procedures in KHPO for the treatment of risk factors for knee OA. MAP = Medial Abrasion Phenomenon; LCP = Lateral Compression Phenomenon; AMR = Arthroscopic Medial Release (since 2000); ACRFP = Arthroscopic Cartilage Regeneration Facilitating Procedure (since 2004); KHPO = Knee Health Promotion Option (since 2007).

Chapter 6

Chapter 6 Knee OA Treatments: The Conventional Protocol vs the KHPO Protocol

The **conventional OA knee treatment protocol** refers to the prevailing standard protocol that bounds virtually all healthcare providers, including members of such dominant standards bodies as the American Academy of Orthopaedic Surgeon (AAOS), the Osteoarthritis Research Society International (OARSI), and European League Against Rheumatism (EULAR).

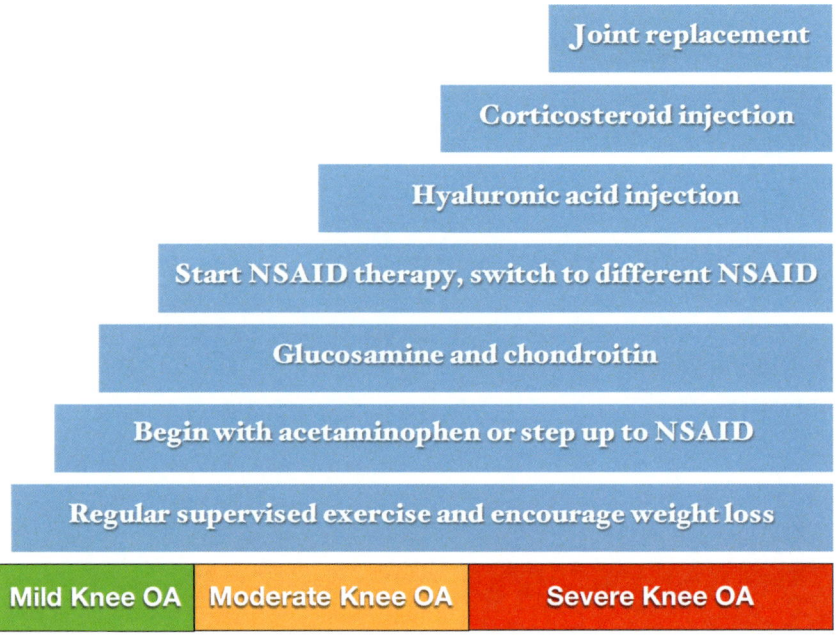

Chapter 6

The KHPO alternative protocol refers to the standard that my practice has developed and utilised since 2007.

Knee Health Promotion Option (KHPO) Protocol

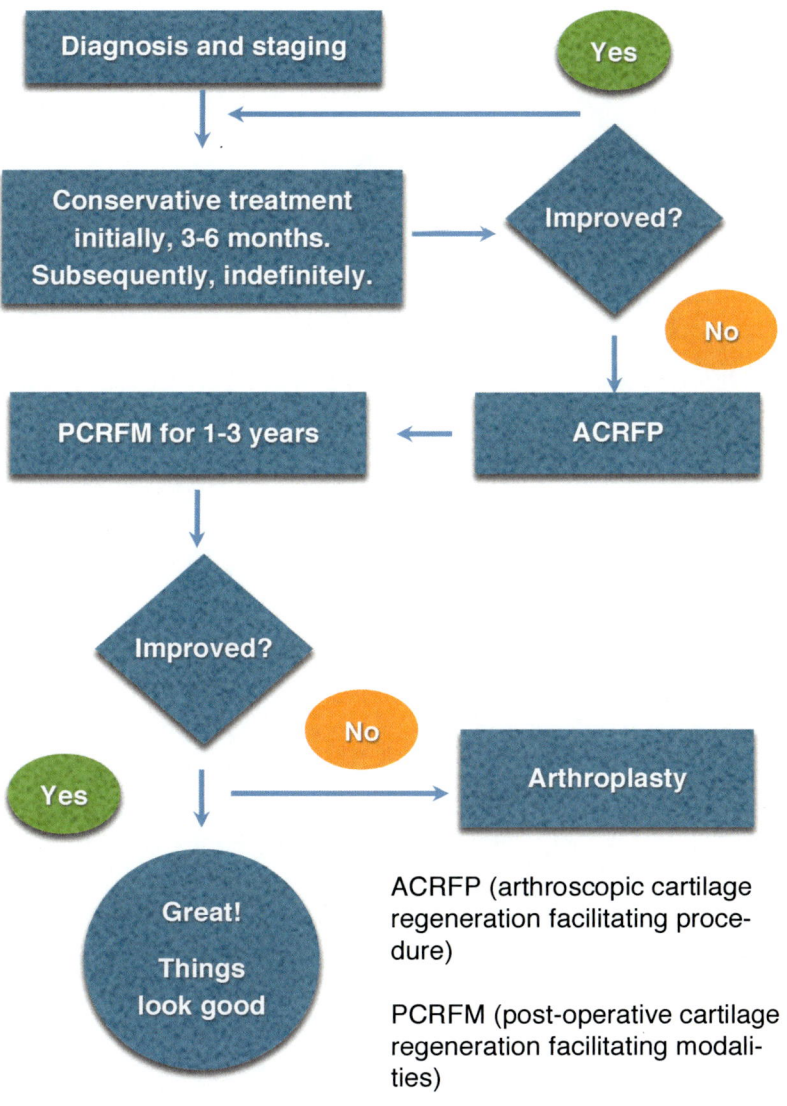

Chapter 6

Food for thought

In my practice, one in four operations that I perform for knee OA patients is knee replacement. The other three are ACRFP, an arthroscopic procedure under the KHPO protocol, which (1) leaves the knee intact but (2) takes out the medial abrasion phenomenon—a potential cause for knee OA—and other risk factors that are damaging the knee. The ratio of knee replacement to ACRFP, is 1 to 3.

In contrast, that ratio for all surgeons in Taiwan is 3 to 1, although the arthroscopic surgery they perform is markedly different from the ACRFP that I perform (see Chapter 5 for why the ACRFP is distinctly better than "their" arthroscopic procedures). Their ineffective arthroscopic procedures have forced them to resort to knee replacements, hence their high knee replacement to arthroscopy ratio.

Orthopaedic surgeons in other countries, like their opposite numbers in Taiwan, also shun arthroscopy as a treatment for knee OA. In fact, they are even more arthroscopy-shy, by a long shot. A recent study points out that only 20% of orthopaedic surgeons worldwide still use arthroscopy to treat knee OA. "Arthroscopic surgery for knee osteoarthritis? Just say no", argue Doctors Anne Mounsey and Bernard Ewigman. [The arthroscopy all of them oppose is not the same as the ACRFP that this book talks about; see **Chapter 5** for a side-by-side comparison. However, because they are not aware of the ACRFP, they are not likely to perform it.] If orthopaedic surgeons throughout the world do not use arthroscopy, their only surgical option to treat knee OA is knee replacement.

So, the doctor you choose to treat your knee OA significantly determines whether you keep your knees or not, statistically speaking.

With the ACRFP, the patients keep their knees, lose their pain, regain function, and get their lives back from their debilitating knee OA.

Let us look at the state of medicine with each protocol.

Chapter 6

The state of conventional treatment protocol for knee OA

Despite the vast amounts of resources that the conventional medical establishment has invested in research, the generally recommended treatment under the conventional protocol for knee OA **has not changed materially for several decades**. In other words, they have not made material progress, much less breakthroughs, in the treatment of knee OA in all those decades. It surely looks like a stagnant protocol, but this is the protocol that healthcare providers follow to treat their patients suffering from knee OA, so most patients anywhere in the world are treated under this conventional protocol.

Essentially, if the symptoms are severe enough and the patient is willing, the surgeon performs a total knee replacement surgery. However, if the symptoms are not severe enough or the patient is unwilling to undergo a total knee replacement, the doctor prescribes **conservative treatments to control the pain, but not at all to remove the underlying cause of knee OA. They cannot remove the underlying cause because they do not know what that cause is.**

Conservative treatments may include rehabilitation exercises, pain medications, glucosamine, chondroitin, intra-articular injections, such as hyaluronic acid and PRP (platelet-rich plasma).

This phase of treatment may last a long time, sometimes several years or even a decade or longer. During this time, the patient likely lives with pain, discomfort, and restricted mobility, and—you guessed it—the affected knee may continue to deteriorate. This deterioration may actually accelerate if the natural protection mechanism—pain—is blocked or tampered with by medication or other ineffective conservative treatments.

In all of these conservation treatments, no action is aimed at eradicating the cause of knee OA. Therefore, patients have no hope of getting better while waiting for knee replacement surgery. The patient goes from waiting

Chapter 6

in pain straight to knee replacement surgery with nothing in between except long days and months of living with pain.

When the damage in the knee is so great as to require knee replacement, then it is done and the knee is irrevocably gone. This is a typical treatment cycle under the conventional protocol.

Chapter 6

The state of KHPO treatment protocol for knee OA

The KHPO is a much better alternative to the foregoing conventional treatment.

We have treated patients under the KHPO protocol since 2007 with remarkably good results. An anecdotal proof of its success is the long waiting list for our service in both outpatient clinics and operating rooms; often they wait for two years for their KHPO surgeries, for example. A more formal proof will be presented below.

The KHPO arthroscopy (ACRFP) removes risk factors for knee OA, and consequently patients, thousands of them, have again become functional, medicine-free, and pain-free, and **most (9 out of 10) of them do not need knee replacements**. Many of them are cured of knee OA.

I know that many of my patients of knee OA firmly believe that the KHPO treatment has saved them from knee replacements and that it has also relieved their knee pains. If they had not heard about and received the KHPO treatment, they would likely have their knees replaced because knee replacement is what the AAOS guidelines call for. These guidelines are very influential, and they are followed by most orthopaedic surgeons.

However, **for all its effectiveness, the KHPO treatment is not yet included in these guidelines.** Please see the following **Patient Activism Chapter (Chapter 7)** for a story about a similar treatment guideline.

Chapter 6

A surgeon's choice and recommendation

"We surgeons tend to do what we are good at doing. If we are good at knee replacement, we do them (to the exclusion of other therapies)", commented a surgeon who took the KHPO clinical training that I taught.

I perform the ACRFP very well. After all, I designed it.

I also do equally well all the things that conventional surgeons can do for their patients, such as knee replacement and all the other procedures in the conventional repertoire. After all, I had been a conventional surgeon myself for many years before I switched to the KHPO. And I still perform knee replacement surgeries for those patients who really need them.

I have practiced under both protocols long enough to know both very well. I perform the ACRFP and the conventional surgeries with equal ease.

Technically, I do not prefer the one to the other, but **conscientiously, I prefer the ACRFP to knee replacement because I believe that the ACRFP is the most beneficial for patient even though this choice means less income for my hospital and for me personally.**

The ACRFP does not preclude knee replacements or any other therapies, if they are called for in the future. In other words, if ACRFP works, you keep your knees, or else if ACRFP fails, you can still have knee replacements. Knee replacement operations are still my favourites when they are called for.

While nobody can predict with certainty whether KHPO will help you or not, the aggregate results of the thousands patients that we have treated under the KHPO tell us that most of them have experienced relief from knee pains and enjoyed improved pain-free mobility and quality of life. They may never need to have knee replacements, and the three KHPO-prescribed daily rehab exercises really help keep their knees in shape to give them extra years of service.

Chapter 6

The KHPO idea is simple, less invasive, and prudent: Treat your knees first with a less invasive, arthroscopic procedure (ACRFP). If it works, as it has worked well for thousands of my patients, good for you. If and only if it does not work, you can always try knee replacement then, and even then you still likely have postponed that dreaded, invasive, and last-resort treatment (knee replacement) by a few years.

And many people find that much more palatable.

Chapter 6

Conventional treatment or the KHPO?

> Would you rather be treated under
> *the conventional treatment protocol* for knee OA?
>
> Under the conventional protocol, you take pain medications, suffer restricted mobility, undergo conservative treatments but do nothing to eradicate the cause of knee OA. So you allow that cause to slowly but inexorably injure your knee, and all you can do is wait hopelessly, sometimes for years, for knee replacement. Conservative treatments may include rehabilitation exercises, pain medications, glucosamine, chondroitin, and intra-articular injections such as hyaluronic acid or PRP (platelet-rich plasma). Since these treatments do not remove any of the risk factors for knee OA, *they cannot be expected to cure the disease*.
>
> Or would you rather be treated under *the KHPO treatment protocol* for knee OA?
>
> Under the KHPO protocol, you intervene early, using arthroscopy to take out all risk factors of knee OA, and, chances are good, you regain function, become pain-free and medicine-free, and avert knee replacement.
>
> *They are your knees, and what you do to protect them is your choice.*

Chapter 6

Now let's take a look at the KHPO

KHPO treatment results: three years after the surgery (Table 3)

Between April 2010 and March 2011, I performed the ACRFP under the KHPO protocol to treat 317 knee OA patients (536 knees). Of them, 286 patients with 480 treated knees have returned for follow-ups at one-, three-, six-month, 1-, 2-, and 3-year after surgery (a 90% follow-up rate). Female/male: 4/1. Age range: 27 – 86 (average 65 years). Most (95.2%, except 10 stage III and 13 stage IV) of these treated knees were still intact three years after surgery.

After they finished their 3-year follow-up, we asked them how they felt about their knees. This is what they told us:

Table 3.

Outcomes of 317 knee OA patients (536 knees) 3 years after the ACRFP

Stage	Knees	Excellent	Good	Fair	Poor	Satisfied
II	195	133 (68.2%)	52 (26.7%)	10 (5.1%)	0	94%
III	216	120 (55.6%)	69 (31.9%)	17 (7.9%)	10 (4.6%)	87.5%
IV	69	30 (43.5%)	25 (36.2%)	1 (1.4%)	13 (18.8%)	79.7%
Total	480	283 (59.0%)	146 (30.4%)	28 (5.8%)	23 (4.8%)	89.4%

Stage = OA staging; Knees = Number of knees; Excellent = greatly improved; Good = apparently improved; Fair = not improved; Poor = worsened; **Satisfied = Excellent + Good (improved)**

Chapter 6

> ***Observation one.*** According to the conventional, mainstream treatment protocol, all 69 stage IV OA knees would have been subjected to the only treatment choice: total knee replacement. Instead, I treated these knees with the ACRFP, and 56 of them are still intact, and they have not been replaced at least three years after the ACRFP. Those original natural knees are still providing useful service to their owners. This alone is extremely good news for the patients and a shot in the arm for me.
>
> ***Observation two.*** Earlier-stage OA knees have enjoyed higher satisfaction rates. The earlier an OA knee is treated with the ACRFP, the better the patient is satisfied with the result. Early treatment is of the essence.

This runs right in the face of the standard conventional treatment protocol—guided by the traditional, stagnant, and outdated knowledge about knee OA—(a) does not recommend active intervention to remove potential pathogenesis of knee OA and (b) allows the disease to progress unchecked until total knee replacement is absolutely required, at which time even the ACRFP cannot probably help them.

It is in a way understandable for the conventional protocol to take that passive stance because, unlike our KHPO protocol, the mainstream medicine currently has not identified a definitive cause for knee OA.

They don't know the cause, so they can't possibly treat it.

Chapter 6

Links about the KHPO

- Official Webpage of Knee Health Promotion Option (KHPO):

    http://www.joint.idv.tw/eng/index.html

- e-Learning Course of Medial Abrasion Syndrome (MAS):

    http://cms.tzuchi.com.tw/dl/DNPTM008EN/player.html

- Water inspiration (medial abrasion syndrome - a cause of knee OA):

    https://www.youtube.com/watch?v=_QRw9pQrgS0

- A Brief Report of New Hope of Knee Osteoarthritis:

    http://www.joint.idv.tw/eng/file/New_Hope_of_Knee_Osteoarthritis.pdf

- Professional Learning Course for KHPO:

    http://www.joint.idv.tw/plc_en/

Chapter 7 Patient Activism

This is a book about knee OA, but please allow me to digress and share with you a story from National Public Radio (NPR) about cancer.

It is a story about how a group of lung cancer survivors changed the established treatment guidelines from the National Comprehensive Cancer Network (NCCN).

The NCCN guidelines are important because oncologists often refer to them first when they are trying to develop treatment plans for their patients.

A group of lung cancer survivors discovered that these guidelines did not include a treatment option that they believed had saved their own lives. **This omission shows that the guidelines do not always reflect newer treatment options.** Some patients might miss out on the benefit of these newer treatment options.

Therefore, **they set out to change the guidelines**. In a sense, these lay people were trying to suggest how, of all people, oncologists should treat lung cancer.

When a type of advanced non-small cell lung cancer has metastasised, it is diagnosed as stage IV. Patients whose cancer has spread are often offered chemotherapy or supportive care rather than surgery or radiation to remove the tumours on the assumption that it is too late to prevent further spread. But some research suggests that patients with oligometastases, or a limited number of spread-out tumours (fewer than three or five, depending on whom you ask) may get significant benefit from more aggressive treatment. **That possibility wasn't reflected in the NCCN guidelines.**

To make a long story short, a group of cancer survivors, led by Chris Newman of Los Molinos, California, submitted a proposal to NCCN just before its guidelines were up for their annual review.

Chapter 7

And when the updated guidelines were released, they included some suggestions from the Newman group. One key phrase from the revision, which took effect January 1, 2015, was: "Aggressive local therapy may be appropriate for selected patients with limited-site oligometastatic disease."

Chris Newman calls the change she helped made to lung cancer treatment guidelines a "small, but very important victory."

"Newman says she's usually pretty cynical about the ability of an individual or small group of patients to make a difference, but that this victory has changed her thinking. 'It's motivated all of us as far as being able to make a difference,' she says. Now she and her fellow patients are each considering what other changes they might push for."

You may visit: http://www.npr.org/sections/health-shots/2015/03/01/385995084/how-a-group-of-lung-cancer-survivors-got-doctors-to-listen to read or listen to the story.

How is this story relevant to knee OA?
Patients may or may not know about all the science behind the treatment that they receive, but they—better than physicians or scientists—do know whether or not that treatment is effective, regardless of whether or not it has been so-called scientifically and statistically proven.

In this sense, this cancer story seems very relevant to the KHPO (knee health promotion **option**), a new, effective, but not yet widely accepted treatment for knee OA. In the same way that Chris Newman knew some of her fellow cancer sufferers were missing out on an effective but not-recommended treatment, I know that knee OA sufferers are missing out on the very real and reliable benefit of pain relief and function recover from the KHPO. They are missing out because, for all its effectiveness, the KHPO is not yet included in the treatment protocols that standards academies have published. Therefore, **healthcare providers are either unaware of or unwilling to try the KHPO.**

Chapter 7

Let me adapt the Chris Newman story to show a point:

Disease	Lung Cancer	Knee OA
Treatment guideline publisher	National Comprehensive Cancer Network (NCCN)	The American Academy of Orthopaedic Surgeons (AAOS)
Old guideline	"chemotherapy or supportive care rather than surgery or radiation"	Knee OA patients should "participate in self-management programs, strengthening, low-impact aerobic exercises, and neuromuscular education; and engage in physical activity consistent with national guidelines"
A consequence of the old guideline	A patient misses out on "a treatment option that they [a group of lung cancer survivors, including Chris Newman and her group] believed had saved their lives"	Patients may lose their knees to knee replacement because they miss out on the ACRFP, an arthroscopic treatment under the KHPO that has relieved knee pains, restored mobility, staved off knee replacement, and kept the knees of thousands of knee OA sufferers.

Chapter 7

Disease	Lung Cancer	Knee OA
Champion of a patient petition to change treatment guidelines	Chris Newman of Los Molinos, California	?
New guideline	In 2015, "Aggressive local therapy may be appropriate for selected patients with limited-site oligometastatic disease."	If this petition is successful, an ideal new guideline may include this: "arthroscopic removal of risk factors that may cause knee OA or injure knee cartilage."

For all its effectiveness, the KHPO treatment is still not yet included in these guidelines.

We are offering this KHPO approach for you, knee pain sufferers, to consider and to talk to your doctors to see whether or not the KHPO approach is right for you. **The KHPO is not included in the established treatment guidelines. But simply because a treatment is not recommended by a treatment guideline does not mean that treatment is not effective. Just ask Chris Newman.**

**Your doctor, and not this book,
will advise you to do what is best for you.**

Chapter 8 A Concerned Surgeon and His Thoughts

I have been a surgeon since 1983. I became an orthopaedic surgeon in 1990, and I have specialised in knee surgery since 2000.

In my orthopaedic practice, I mainly treat patients who suffer from knee OA. Each month, I usually see 100 referred patients with knee OA, for whom the initial course of action usually includes non-invasive measures under the guideline of KHPO. For some patients (around 30 of them), those are all the treatment they ever need to regain their freedom of movement and quality of life, but for the others (around 70 of them) whose pain persists, invasive therapies including ACRFP (around 50 of them) and arthroplasty (around 20 of them) become necessary.

When non-invasive measures are unable to provide relief, most orthopaedic surgeons, following the conventional treatment protocol, will perform either a partial or a total knee replacement. However, because either type is non-reversible, knee replacement should only be considered when all other options have been tried and failed. Knee replacement is an irrevocable last resort; it is a serious decision.

I have tried to help my patients avoid knee replacement by offering them the ACRFP, a potent and effective arthroscopic alternative to the non-reversible open surgery of partial or total knee replacement.

Since 2004, I have suggested to thousands of suitable patients to undergo the ACRFP under the KHPO protocol as an alternative to knee replacement, which most surgeons under conventional treatment protocols would have advised. Consequently, my pa-

Chapter 8

tients have kept their knees, regained pain-free mobility, and reclaimed their lives from knee OA.

I need to stress again that I perform knee replacement operations and ACRFP with equal ease, and I have successfully and regularly done both types of surgery in my practice. I do not personally prefer the one to the other in my recommendation to my patients, but I do prefer to recommend the procedure that I believe is the least invasive possible and yet most effective in relieving their pain and keeping their knees, taking into full account of their individual conditions.

I have tried hard to help my patients keep their knees with the ACRFP despite the fact that performing knee replacement operations would have been a path of less resistance for me to take. After all, knee replacement is a widely accepted procedure that the established treatment protocols have called for. In contrast, the ACRFP is a new kid on the block, which few orthopaedic surgeons know about, much less embrace.

I could very well simply follow that conventional protocol and do knee replacements for my patients. Then I would not raise any eyebrows, I would have better income, and my patients would in most cases experience quicker relief than they could from the ACRFP—in the short run.

But, in the long run, knee replacement recipients face risks such as potential infections or worn prosthesis while people who receive ACRFP can regain function, return to pain-free mobility, and keep their knees. This is why I cannot just "go with the flow" of the conventional protocol and recommend knee replacement; I will not do a knee replacement when the ACRFP can relieve knee pain and keep the knees for a patient, any patient.

I have been quite successful in my pursuit of helping my patients keep their knees. It is quite heartening to just think of this fact.

Chapter 8

Knee replacement vs ACRFP

Let us compare knee replacement and the ACRFP from three perspectives: (1) the invasiveness of the surgery and its damage to the body, (2) what if the procedure fails, and (3) the situation in a few years after the procedure.

(1) **Knee replacement is much more invasive and complicated**, involving more than 100 steps. The complexity of a knee replacement surgery can clearly be seen from the myriad of tools needed for the procedure:

    (a) scalpels,

    (b) retractors to keep the large incision open during surgery,

    (c) surgical saw, drills, chisel, hammer, curettes and bone files to remove the surfaces of diseased or damaged joint, to shape the underlying bone to exactly fit the metal and plastic components of the artificial knee,

    (d) angle measurement instruments to ensure that all alignments are exactly right to allow smooth motion of the knee, and

    (e) bone cement, bone cement mixing bowl, bone cement delivery gun, to glue the man-made parts on the patella, the femur, and the tibia.

These tools are remarkably like those needed to remodel a house.

Open surgery is needed for knee replacement. In contrast, **the ACRFP is a minimally invasive because it needs only four small incisions for the insertion of arthroscopic instruments**.

(2) **If a knee replacement fails, the patient has no alternative treatment**, yet the real knee is gone, and there is no going back. The only remedial action is a revision surgery to put in a larger prosthesis to replace the failed prosthesis.

Chapter 8

If an ACRFP fails, the patient has recourse: The patient can still have his or her diseased knee replaced.

(3) **An artificial knee is subject to wear just as a natural knee is**, but there is a significant difference between the two. An artificial knee does not regenerate and does not have the ability to repair itself, but your own knee does. Moreover, an artificial knee does not have normal blood circulation to protect itself from invasive bacteria, nor can it ward off infection.

Therefore, if a knee replacement has failed due to wear or infection, the patient goes through another invasive knee replacement again. The procedure is to clean out the broken implants, possibly repeat debridement surgery for the infection, and put in a bigger prosthesis. After the surgery, the patient goes through tough recovery and all the rehabilitation programs all over again.

Even after all this trouble and suffering, the patient is usually less satisfied with the replacement prosthesis than the original one. The new device that the revision surgery puts in usually functions less satisfactorily than the primary one.

Conversely, a patient treated with ACRFP may never need to have his or her knee surgically treated again. The ACRFP may be the last surgery they need to relieve their knee OA pains.

Most of our ACRFP patients have kept their natural knees, walked pain free and return to their healthy lives. If the ACRFP is not effective for some patients, they can then receive knee replacement—and they got to keep their knees a while longer.

Given the above comparison, conscience and the pursuit of a viable treatment option compel me to go down the lonely path of the ACRFP.

I write this book to share the ACRFP with patients who have not had the opportunity to learn about it or benefit from it. Many knee OA sufferers have benefited from it, maybe you can, too.

Chapter 9 Evidence-based Medicine Part I: Patients' Choices

Evidence-based medicine (EBM), or evidence-based practice (EBP) includes:

- **Best scientific evidence**
- **Physicians' clinical experiences**
- **Patients' choices**

Here, I will present to you EBM as it applies to the treatment of knee OA. Working our way backward, let's start with patients' choices, with the testimonials of some of the patients whom I treated under the KHPO protocol.

Let me repeat some stats (Table 3) to set the stage for their testimonials:

Chapter 9

Table 3. Between April 2010 and March 2011, I treated 317 patients (536 knees) with the ACRFP under the concept of KHPO. Of them, 286 patients with 480 treated knees have returned for follow-ups at one-, three-, six-month, 1-, 2-, and 3-year after surgery (a 90% follow-up rate after 3 years). Female/male: 4/1. Age range: 27 – 86 (average 65 years)

Stage	Knees	Excellent	Good	Fair	Poor	Satisfied
II	195	133 (68.2%)	52 (26.7%)	10 (5.1%)	0	94%
III	216	120 (55.6%)	69 (31.9%)	17 (7.9%)	10 (4.6%)	87.5%
IV	69	30 (43.5%)	25 (36.2%)	1 (1.4%)	13 (18.8%)	79.7%
Total	480	283 (59.0%)	146 (30.4%)	28 (5.8%)	23 (4.8%)	89.4%

Stage = OA staging; Knees = Number of knees; Excellent = greatly improved; Good = apparently improved; Fair = not improved; Poor = worsened; Satisfied = Excellent + Good (improved)

ACRFP under the KHPO protocol has achieved success. With it, thousands of patients have consequently enjoyed improved quality of life and freedom of movement. Some of them share their stories. Most stories were written at least two or three years after the ACRFP, time enough for them to give their own knees an assessment.

Each of these patients would most likely have been a recipient of artificial knees if I had not treated them with the ACRFP under the concept of KHPO. In short, each of them has kept their knees as a direct result of the ACRFP. In fact, if you read from their own words, the ACRFP has cured their knee OA, and many of them, with their knees working so well, may never need to have knee replacement. Here are their stories. At the risk of making a long chapter, I have largely not abbreviated their letters so you may get a more complete picture of their states of mind several years after being treated with ACRFP.

Chapter 9

Testimonial 1: Give yourself a chance

Last name: Chen, male, knee OA stage III. Age at the bilateral ACRFP treatment in March 2011: 65.

A business owner, Mr. Chen started his daily exercise regimen of morning lap swimming, 5k jogging, and golfing when he was 37, and he stayed with it for almost 30 years.

He began to feel knee pain a few years ago. He sought help from orthopaedic surgeons at three medical centers. The first surgeon suggested knee replacement. Mr. Chen sought a second opinion and then a third. The last two surgeons agreed with the first.

Despite their anonymous opinion, Mr. Chen was not ready to have parts of his body replaced by artificial devices, so he checked around some more.

A friend told him about the ACRFP (arthroscopic cartilage regeneration facilitating procedure) that a Dr. Shaw-Ruey Lyu has been doing for many patients, so he took a trip to southern Taiwan to see the doctor.

Dr. Lyu advised Mr. Chen that he had stage III knee OA, and ACRFP(arthroscopic cartilage regeneration facilitating procedure) under the concept of KHPO (knee health promotion option) was a suitable treatment for him. He was scheduled to return nine months later for the surgery due to the long waiting list. It would be a long wait, but he liked the fact that (1) the ACRFP, an arthroscopic procedure with small incisions, was not too invasive, (2) he would keep his knees, (3) the Joint Center at Dalin Tzu Chi Hospital had successfully treated numerous patients like him over the years, and (4) Dr. Lyu's professionalism during his clinic visit had won his complete trust. Therefore, he decided to wait patiently for his turn.

As scheduled, Dr. Lyu performed the ACRFP on Mr. Chen in March 2011, after which he took pain medications for only a week. He has not needed to take any more of them ever since.

Chapter 9

One week after the surgery, he managed to walk slowly up to his living room on the second floor, and he was able to take care of himself without constraints. He has been quite satisfied with the surgery on both knees, and he has been a stickler for the three rehabilitation exercises, which he has consistently done at home every day. He has followed the directions of the medical team without fail.

He was also quick to acknowledge that the rehab had not always been a cinch. In fact, in the early days of his recovery, his knees had hurt so badly during rehab that he had several times considered giving up or skipping a few days. Luckily, he has never allowed these thoughts to get the better of him. Since his initial appointment with Dr. Lyu, Mr. Chen has been convinced of the critical importance of the three daily rehab exercises.

He knows that Dr. Lyu and his team have done their part to fix his knees, and it is now his turn to carry out his part of the bargain if he wants to reap the maximum benefit from the surgery. Mr. Chen has walked an hour and done the three rehab exercises every day. Predictably, the pain has diminished with time, and he has returned to Dr. Lyu's clinic for follow-ups as scheduled. The X-rays of his knees at two years after the surgery clearly showed that the joint space between his bones was wider than before the surgery and that there were signs of cartilage regeneration inside his knees.

His recovery has been satisfactory and getting better. He is confident about his knees.

"A patient must trust the medical team. After the doctor has surgically removed the primary causes of your knee OA, you have to do the rehab exercises every day forever. You cannot stop that regimen, not even when it hurts during the exercise," Mr. Chen advised those who would soon be operated on and those who are recovering from the same surgery that he had gotten from Dr. Lyu.

"Give your body a chance," he urged them earnestly. "Please have confidence in yourself."

Chapter 9

Testimonial 2: Improved quality of life

Ms. Huang, 67, stage III and IV knee OA, bilateral ACRFP in early 2011.

She used to have aches and pains here and there after doing too many chores. She paid no heed, assuming she had joint degeneration that came with ageing. But her knee pain worsened so much that she could no longer stand it, and she had difficulties moving about and standing for long periods of time. It was only then when she realised that something was very wrong, and she began seeing the doctors.

At the community hospital near her home, she was told that the cartilage in both of her knees was severely worn, and she was advised to have knee replacements as soon as possible. But she thought that such an invasive treatment should be saved as a last resort, and she asked herself what would happen if knee replacements should fail. It was frightening to think about the worst-case scenario, so she hesitated.

In the meantime, the doctor prescribed pain and muscle relaxing medications. They did deliver temporary relief. However her knee pain would return as soon as she stopped the drugs. Furthermore, Ms. Huang had a bad kidney, and she knew all too well the damage that taking medicine for long periods of time might do to her kidneys. She knew that she could not rely on pain medications forever.

Huang had a friend who had been treated with ACRFP (arthroscopic cartilage regeneration facilitating procedure). He shared his ACRFP experiences with her. Huang suddenly saw a glimmer of hope for her knees.

Dalin Tzu Chi Hospital hosted a knee health promotion forum in September 2010 in Taipei, which Huang attended. Dr. Shaw-Ruey Lyu explained the causes and his treatment approach for osteoarthritic knees. Huang was thrilled by what she had heard. After the forum, she got on the calendar of Dr. Lyu for a clinic visit three months later at the Dalin Tzu Chi Hospital.

At the clinic, Dr. Lyu informed Huang that her knees had stages III and IV OA, respectively, and that both knees could be treated with the ACRFP.

Chapter 9

The stage-IV knee might not recover as well as the stage-III knee would. Ms. Huang decided right then and there to have ACRFP done on both of her knees.

She really wanted to have the procedure done sooner rather than later, but the queue for Dr. Lyu's surgery was very long. She decided to take advantage of the less congested surgery calendars during the Chinese New Year holidays to have Dr. Lyu perform ACRFP on her knees. Most Taiwanese patients avoid having surgery during that time. She would have had to wait much longer at other times of year.

After the surgery, she conscientiously did the rehab exercises every day exactly as directed by Dr. Lyu's team. She returned for follow-ups exactly as scheduled as well. Her X-rays at one year post op showed cartilage regeneration in both knees.

She has done the suggested rehab exercises every day without fail since her surgery more than two years ago. Except the few days immediately following the surgery, she has not taken any medications or probiotics for her knees. She has, however, frequently taken sightseeing tours overseas. It is her opinion that the improved quality of life has made her surgery by Dr. Lyu most worthwhile.

"Before the surgery, I could not even make it to the market for grocery, and my life was miserable. But now I'm able to go wherever I want and whenever I please. I'm back to normal," she said. Certain movements require special attention. "You should slow down in squatting down and standing up so that you won't put sudden and excessive pressure on the knees. Likewise for walking up or down the stairs," she advised. She is confident that she has gotten the hang of taking care of her own knees.

Chapter 9

Testimonial 3: Thanks to the KHPO, I can jog again!

Mr. Wu, male, stages III and IV, respectively. Received bilateral ACRFP in November 2010.

"I am thankful for what happened to me on November 4, 2010. On that day, Dr. Lyu performed ACRFP (arthroscopic cartilage regeneration facilitating procedure) on both of my knees. The procedure cured the knee OA that had debilitated me for more than a decade during which I had knee pains, and my mobility was severely curtailed. Now I can walk freely without knee pains, and I enjoy better quality of life. That has been a most memorable day indeed," Mr. Wu said. He is a retired high school biology teacher in Zhudong, Hsinchu in northern Taiwan.

Mr. Wu had had painful knees for more than a decade. He had sought treatment from four orthopaedic surgeons at medical centres, and they separately arrived at the same treatment recommendation: knee replacement.

Mr. Wu thought that knee replacement was more than invasive; it was destructive to the real knee in order to put in the artificial devices. If he proceeded as those surgeons had advised, it would be the end of his knees. There would be no going back. Therefore, he really hesitated. He just could not accept that finality. In the meantime, he continued to look for alternative treatments.

One day in 2010, he read in a newspaper that a team at Dalin Tzu Chi Hospital had pioneered an advanced arthroscopic procedure to treat osteoarthritic knees and that the team had achieved impressive success, helping many patients reclaim their mobility without pain medications and without resorting to knee replacements. Curious, he signed up for a forum on the procedure: the knee health promotion option (KHPO).

In the forum, he heard Dr. Lyu describe a potential cause of osteoarthritic knees and a set of arthroscopic procedures, collectively called the ACRFP

Chapter 9

under the KHPO protocol, to eradicate that cause. Mr. Wu was convinced that this approach was right for him, so he decided to receive the KHPO treatment on both of his knees, then at stages III and IV, respectively. **Dr. Lyu operated on Mr. Wu in November 2010.**

Prior to the surgery, Mr. Wu had difficulty walking, much less running, which he had not been able to do for more than a decade. But after having recovered from the KHPO surgery, he exclaimed one day, "**I was able to start jogging gently in March 2013.**" Mr. Wu has finally regained the freedom of jogging, and he can now experience once again the joy that only jogging can deliver.

"I'm living proof of the wonders of ACRFP. This procedure has enabled cartilage regeneration in my knees, and consequently my knee pain has disappeared," Mr. Wu said. "And my legs have become strong and coordinated enough for me to jog once again. I'm really fortunate." His long struggle with OA knee pain has made him an expert patient in the disease. He has gained a comprehensive understanding of the KHOP and ACRFP concepts, and he can talk freely about them like a professional.

"In retrospect, my choice of the KHPO and Dr. Lyu was great," Mr. Wu said confidently three years after he had received the treatment.

Chapter 9

Testimonial 4: A complete medical team for a sprinter who tried glucosamine and hyaluronic acid shots to no avail

Ms. Zeng is a medical care provider living in Hualien, Eastern Taiwan. She was a sprinter in middle school, and she continued to run explosive sprints after she had started working.

While in her 30s, she began to have severe knee pain. She was diagnosed with chondromalacia patellas, more commonly known as runner's knees, and her doctors advised her to stop running. That marked the beginning of her struggle with knee pain that would last nearly 20 years.

At first, **she used imported glucosamine for eight months**. That was expensive stuff, but her pain did not let up. Then she **followed her doctor's suggestion and got hyaluronic acid injections**. At the time, such injections were not covered by the national health insurance program in Taiwan, and she paid for them out of her own pocket. It was only later that she could apply on a case-by-case basis to the insurer for prior approval to receive these shots. But regardless of who paid for the injections, Ms. Zeng **noticed that she had needed these shots more and more frequently**. Apparently each shot was giving her less and less relief, so she switched to rehabilitation, hoping to get some pain relief.

She and her husband took a pleasure trip to France in 2010. While there, she could not squat down to use the toilet, and she could not stand up from her seat after a two-hour movie. There was no denying that her knees were degrading her quality of life.

Doctors suggested knee replacements, but Ms. Zeng, still so young, could not accept that. She stepped up her research efforts for alternative treatments and gather on-line information on degenerative osteoarthritic knees. She stumbled upon the personal blog of Dr. Shaw-Ruey Lyu.

From the blog, Ms. Zeng learned the science behind the arthroscopic cartilage regeneration facilitating procedure (ACRFP). She also learned that the

Chapter 9

Joint Center at Dalin Tzu Chi Hospital, which Dr. Lyu heads, employs clear and precise procedures before, during, and after the ACRFP surgery for a patient's osteoarthritic knees. She thought that Dr. Lyu's program was truly a godsend. She was thrilled to have finally found a therapy that she had always wanted.

She wanted to see Dr. Lyu, and she did not want to see Dr. Lyu: On the one hand, he and his team, their procedures and expertise, and their success stories were all propelling her their way, but they were also several hundred kilometers from her home in Eastern Taiwan.

She looked very hard for surgeons in Eastern Taiwan who could perform the ACRFP. Her futile search led her to conclude that she had to go to Dr. Lyu, so she went to the Joint Centre at the Dalin Tzu Chi Hospital for the ACRFP.

Ms. Zeng summed it up, "The Joint Centre had successfully treated many patients over many years. Its professional nursing staff, rehab therapists, and surgery team make a complete program that has earned my trust.

"Dr. Lyu's blog shows the results of his research and surgeries. The statistics, scientific evidence, and his papers on international journals all served to convince me to seek treatment from him. It is true that I had to wait a long time in the queue for his surgery, but the result has justified every minute of the wait."

Ms. Zeng has taken several trips to other countries since the surgery more than a year ago. "Once at Huanglong, Sichuan, I was able to follow the group on a trek to higher than 3,000 meters above sea level. I held back to protect my reborn knees, so I was not quite as quick as before," she said.

Chapter 9

Testimonial 5: Six hyaluronic acid injections in vain

Ms. Yang, 83, lives alone in Jiayi, Southern Taiwan. She received bilateral ACRFP in 2010.

Her daughter, Ms. Qian of Kaohsiung, noticed three years ago that her mother walked funny and she fell often. She believed that something was wrong with her mother's legs. She took her to see many doctors in Jiayi and Kaohsiung. With just a few exceptions, all the doctors concluded that her mother was suffering from knee osteoarthritis. She even had an arthroscopy that did not help [not to be confused with the arthroscopic treatments of the ACRFP].

Ms. Qian asked the doctors to perform knee replacements for her mother, but, perhaps because of her old age, none of the doctors was willing to operate on her. Meanwhile, her knee pain got worse, so she paid for six hyaluronic acid injections out of her own pocket. However, the pain did not abate.

Ms. Yang used to be energetic and independent. She used to take care of herself and was active in her social circles, but her knee pain took all that away. Ms. Qian loved her mother, but she could not live with her to care for her. All the futile treatments made the two of them thoroughly frustrated.

Ms. Qian, a Christian, prayed, and she entreated the gods in local temples to help relieve her mother's pain. For her mother's sake, Ms. Qian was willing to do anything, even something as directly at odds with her religious belief as worshiping in a temple. Still, there was no relief for her mother.

One night Ms. Qian was watching TV when she happened to see Dr. Shaw-Ruey Lyu talking about knee osteoarthritis and a novel approach [the arthroscopic medial release (AMR) under the ACRFP] that he had being using for years with great success. Thinking [wrongly] that novel approach

Chapter 9

was the same as the arthroscopic surgery that her mother had been through to no benefit, Ms. Qian paid no heed. But her friends beseeched her to explore, so she took her mother to see Dr. Lyu.

Dr. Lyu shared with them the concept of cartilage regeneration and told them that the first year after surgery would be key to her recovery. The patient must cooperate fully with the medical team and follow all of its directions in order to achieve the expected result. Knowing nothing better to do, they decided to fully comply with Dr. Lyu's directions. "If it fails again, we'll give up," Ms. Qian recalled her desperation.

Ms. Yang received the ACRFP in 2010 on both of her knees. She did the rehab exercises diligently, never slacking off despite the pain, and she showed up for her follow-ups as scheduled. Now her X-rays clearly show wider joint space in both of her knees and regenerated cartilage. She is recovering exactly as expected.

Ms. Yang now lives alone once again, and she lives completely independently. She goes around freely without using any walking aid. Meanwhile, she is still doing her daily rehab routine, never missing a day. Since the surgery, she has never taken any supplements.

"I'm grateful," Ms. Qian said.

Chapter 9

Testimonial 6: High praise for the medical team

Mr. Chen received the ACRFP in 2012.

Unlike most knee OA patients, Mr. Chen of Tainan did not shop around for the best treatment for his painful knees. He went straight to Dr. Shaw-Ruey Lyu because his cardiologist son suggested him to. Dr. Chen helped guide his father through the entire treatment process.

Before he retired, Mr. Chen was a teacher, and his job required him to sit for long periods of time. He played tennis. He began to experience knee pains eight years ago. The pains were particularly pronounced when he took the stairs up or down. Initially, he down-played the pain.

Following his retirement, he took up serious mountaineering. He often trekked up peaks higher than 3,000 meters (just shy of 10,000 feet), of which Taiwan has 275. He experienced extreme knee pains during and after his hikes.

His son, the cardiologist, noticed the deterioration of his knees and recommended that he see Dr. Shaw-Ruey Lyu. Dr. Chen had heard about Dr.Lyu's theory and arthroscopic surgical approach for knee OA, and the success in pain relief that he and his team had achieved for their patients, all without resorting to knee replacements.

Mr. Chen received the ACRFP from Dr. Lyu in 2012. Now more than a year later, he walks ten thousand steps and plays tennis for 30 minutes a day. He does not take any drugs or supplements. Many of his friends suffer osteoarthritic knee pains, so Mr. Chen cheerfully and proudly shares his experiences and success with them. He holds Dr. Lyu and his team at the Joint Center of Dalin Tzu Chi Hospital in high regard.

"After I decided to receive the surgery, I had to wait quiet a long time for my turn. The nurses at the Joint Centre gave me clear and specific before-the-surgery instructions, so I felt quite at ease while waiting at home for the surgery. I knew what the surgery would entail, and I was not scared," Mr.

Chapter 9

Chen said. "During the actual surgery, I clearly saw the culprit of my knee problem on the monitor for the arthroscopy because Dr. Lyu explained to me as he performed the procedure. After the surgery, therapists taught me how to do rehab exercises so I could do them at home.

"During the first year after the surgery, my case specialist kept track of my rehab progress and reminded me to return to the Joint Center for follow-ups. They have got a high-caliber team there. Their approach is really good for their patients. My friends have never had been treated so nicely elsewhere."

Mr. Chen continued, "Each member on Dr. Lyu's team has a specific job to do. They are professional and efficient. Patients completely trust Dr. Lyu and his team. That's why the Joint Center at Dalin Tzu Chi Hospital is so successful."

Mr. Chen does not just share his experience with others. He shares it with his son, Dr. Chen, too. He urges his son to adopt the patient-centric philosophy at the Joint Center and apply it in his own cardiology practice and to spread it to other physicians. Mr. Chen hopes that many more patients can benefit from such philosophy.

Chapter 9

Testimonial 7: Cartilage regenerated

A car accident in 1990 injured the patella in both of Mr. Li's knees when he was just 24 years old. The surgery at the time was less than successful, and he was left to suffer knee pains in the next 20 years. "I couldn't find any reason to live another day," he, now 47, recalls his desperation and agony that his knee pains caused.

After the accident, his knees could only move laterally, so he could not bend his knees much at all. He was forced to remove badminton, once his love and forte, from his life entirely. His knees gave him dull pains, and he was often awakened by sudden spasmodic pains in the middle of his sleep. That was no way to live, but he was too young to concede defeat and give it all up.

He started seeking treatment all over Taiwan, having tried top-tier teaching hospitals and faculty surgeons known for their expertise in knee osteoarthritis. He tried every new type of instrument and every therapeutic technique on the market purporting to relieve knee pains. Whether such treatment was covered by insurance was of no concern to Mr. Li. He just wanted to get his knees back.

In the course of his decade-long search for a cure, he tried arthroscopic surgery several times, but none helped. Several doctors told him that, with his knee cartilage virtually all worn out, his best option was knee replacements. But he knew, from the experiences of his relatives, that **even knee replacements could not always deliver relief** that the patient expected. Therefore, Mr. Li, still quite young, never seriously considered knee replacements.

Teaching in a college, Mr. Li is curious, and the information that he had picked up over the years of treatment had made him almost as knowledgeable about knee structure and diseases as a medical professional. All that knowledge, however, did not lead him to accept the notion that cartilage could not regenerate, which was exactly what most of his surgeons had told him. Only one doctor told him otherwise, suggesting him to get a cartilage

Chapter 9

regenerating transplant. He pointed out to Mr. Li that it might be his only hope. The problem was that no surgeon in Taiwan could perform that procedure for him. He could get the transplant in the United States. Mr. Li did not go for it out of cost considerations.

Mr. Li continued searching for a treatment as his knees continued to pain him.

He found Dr. Shaw-Ruey Lyu's blog in 2011. He was glad to see that Dr. Lyu was also of the opinion that cartilage could regenerate. He got an appointment. At the clinic, Dr. Lyu explained the theory of cartilage regeneration and his approach to surgery in the general scheme of the knee health promotion option, or KHPO. Mr. Li decided to receive the surgery from Dr. Lyu. Even though the first available slot was 18 months hence, Mr. Li waited patiently. Finally the big day came when Dr. Lyu performed the arthroscopic cartilage regenerating facilitating procedure (ACRFP) on both of his knees in April 2013.

It has been over two years since the surgery. Mr. Li has noticed tremendous changes in his knees. Mr. Li sometimes needs to squat down to go to the bathroom. He has been able to stand up from a squatting position much more easily than before. His knees no longer cause him spasmodic pain in the middle of the night. Also his knees are no longer the accurate weather forecasters that they were before the ACRFP; they used to dependably forecast the arrival of temperature changes or spiking humidity.

"Blessedly, my knees seem quite insensitive to the wintery weather this year," Mr. Li said. "The excruciating pains are gone. I'm really surprised by all the pleasant changes."

When asked about the most significant factors that had contributed to the success of his ACRFP, he pointed out (1) the underlying medical theory of the KHPO protocol, (2) precise execution of the protocol, (3) simplicity of the protocol, (4) reasonable costs to patients, and (5) the absence of extended drug use after surgery.

Chapter 9

He went on to say, "Of course, the rehab exercises after the surgery is so important that they directly affect the efficacy of the KHPO treatment. **If a patient does not do the rehab exercises every day as directed, he or she is contributing to the less-than-ideal result. Conversely, if a patient does them diligently every day, then he or she helps to bring about ideal results.**" Mr. Li again emphasised the significance of at-home rehab exercises and their impact on the eventual result of the treatment.

His ACRFP surgery made 2013 a year of abundant blessing for Mr. Li. His mobility and quality of life have improved. He has regained his cheerful spirits and outlook for life. He feels that he is beginning a new phase of his life with full use of his knees.

"I feel a joy of rebirth, something quite beyond words," Mr. Li said. "I'm grateful to Dr. Lyu. I wish that I'd met him sooner."

Chapter 9

Testimonial 8: Father-son pair under the KHPO program—a complete knee health regimen

Mr. Wang had stage III knee OA with all the typical symptoms. A firm believer that body parts should not be removed lightly, he rejected any recommendations of knee replacements, which most of his doctors had made. Therefore, when he learned about the KHPO regimen that Dr. Shaw-Ruey Lyu was practicing at Dalin Tzu Chi Hospital, he quickly and confidently scheduled for the service. He has been more than pleased with how his knees have improved since the ACRFP under the KHPO.

Mr. Wang has a 42-year-old son, a mechanical engineer. On the job, he often needed to carry 20 kilograms (44 pounds) of equipment up and down the stairs. His knees had long been overburdened. His own weight, approaching 100 kilograms (220 pounds) did not help matters. One day in 2011, the son collapsed on the floor at work because his knees gave out. Given his father's favourable outcome, he went straight to Dr. Lyu.

The cartilage in his knees was severely worn, and Dr. Lyu suggested ACRFP. He took advantage of a surgery slot that had opened up because another patient had canceled because of superstition. He was therefore fast-tracked. Dr. Lyu operated on him in April 2012.

As with all patients in the KHPO program, Mr. Wang's treatment had started the moment he stepped into Dr. Lyu's clinic. Based on his conditions, Dr. Lyu's team suggested to him specific helpful things that he could do at home or at work while waiting for surgery. Those things were tailored for him and were designed to put him in a position to avoid further damage by the medial abrasion phenomenon and to get the most benefit from the upcoming ACRFP.

The team advised him to do exercises to strengthen his quadriceps, to use knee braces, to avoid careless or repeated bending of his knees, and to minimise the weight that he would carry on the job in order to slow the deterioration of his knees while awaiting surgery. He took all their advice to heart and executed them diligently.

Chapter 9

After surgery, his father, now an old hand, supervised and guided him in his post-operative care and rehabilitation exercises. He has thoroughly done what he needs to do—the rehab exercises—every day ever since surgery.

One year after surgery, his knee X-rays showed signs of cartilage regeneration. They also showed that joint space had opened up in his knee. His life has returned to normal at home and at work, exactly as expected.

"Like Dad, I like to keep my body parts intact, and I don't like foreign objects in my body. Less invasive treatments are better and are the preferred choice for patients," Mr. Wang, the engineer, said of his choice of the KHPO over knee replacements.

Chapter 9

Testimonial 9: At 90+, she's still active and going places 10 years after the ACRFP.

A physician professor helped his mother choose the ACRFP, which she received when she was in her 80s.

Dr. Li Cheng-hua, deputy director-general, National Health Insurance Administration, Ministry of Health and Welfare, wrote the following on June 22, 2014.

Ten years ago [in 2004], a medical school professor at a national university in Taipei [where the very best hospitals in the nation were clustered] drove his 80-something mother nearly 200 miles to a rural town in southern Taiwan. He checked her into the orthopaedic ward at Dalin Tzu Chi Hospital.

The next morning, Dr. Shaw-Ruey Lyu performed an arthroscopic cartilage regeneration facilitating procedure (ACRFP) on her. Two days later, the professor checked his mother out and drove her back to her home in Taipei. She did her daily rehabilitation exercises as Dr. Lyu had directed. Soon she was able to stay out of bed and walk without [her age-old knee] pain. Three weeks after surgery, she was able to walk normally, and she started her daily routine of walking to neighbourhood markets to buy grocery for the day, a routine of many work-at-home Taiwanese housewives. She also takes leisurely walks every afternoon to a nearby park and catch up on the latest with her neighbours and friends. She has regained her mobility, resumed normal activities, and reclaimed her quality of life.

I know this woman well. [I am that med school professor.] She is my mother. She suffered in her 80s from serious osteoarthritis of the knees. I immediately thought of "Wei-Ming in the north and Shaw-Ruey in the south," two outstanding orthopaedic surgeons, Dr. Wei-Ming Chen of Taipei Veteran General Hospital in northern Taiwan, and Dr. Shaw-Ruey Lyu of Dalin Tzu Chi Hospital in the south. Their excellence has won them patients' appreciation far and wide.

Chapter 9

Dr. Lyu directs the joint center at his hospital. [While an expert in the full range of treatment for knee pain,] he has focused on knee osteoarthritis and developed a novel treatment regimen that [without going into details] employs arthroscopic surgeries to cure the knee pain of most of his patients [of which he has thousands]. They therefore never need to have knee replacement surgery.

While either of these two doctors would have been an excellent first choice to treat my mother, she was quite old at the time, and she did not want to undergo a major surgery like knee replacement. Therefore, I braved the 400-mile drive and took my mother to see Dr. Lyu.

Many people are afflicted with osteoarthritis of the knee. In the course of treating many such patients over the decades, Dr. Lyu has observed closely and amassed a wealth of clinical data on the disease. He has found that fibrous medial plica tend to quicken the abrasion and degeneration of knee cartilage. **He has devised a novel arthroscopic procedure [called the ACRFP] to remove the inflamed tissues and adjust the tension between parts of the knee structure. The objective is to ease the painful symptoms and to provide an environment that is more hospitable to the cure and regeneration of damaged cartilage.**

The ACRFP can delay or even make it unnecessary to have knee replacement surgery. It is a superior treatment option for patients suffering from knee osteoarthritis. My mother talked this matter over with me, a physician, and then she decided to go for the ACRFP.

It has been ten years since my mother's ACRFP treatment by Dr. Lyu. Thanks to his treatment, my mother, even in her 90s now, still walks around freely, independently, and without pain. She still enjoys herself. She and I would love to tell the world how wonderful that ACRFP has been.

Chapter 9

Testimonial 10: Three couples, four ACRFPs

Three couples live near a school in a Taipei suburb. They often run into each other on their morning walks around the campus, so they often talk together about their retirement lives, occasionally bragging about how well their knees are holding up. Turns out that the group has another thing in common: Four of them have received the ACRFP treatment from Dr. Shaw-Ruey Lyu for their knee pain, so at least one spouse in each couple has been his patient.

Mr. A ran a timberland and paper mill business in Vietnam, so for a long time he used to climb mountains and bear heavy loads. These two risk factors for knee osteoarthritis did consequently lead him to suffer severely from this disease. Word of mouth led him to see Dr. Lyu, who performed the ACRFP on him in **March 2012**. He recovered quite nicely. One year after surgery, he suggested that his wife, Mrs. A, also a long-time sufferer of the same disease, receive the ACRFP, too.

Mr. and Mrs. A live in the same community as Mr. and Mrs. B. Mrs. A and Mrs. B often ran into each other at the community hot spring. Mrs. A noticed that Mrs. B seemed to walk with difficulty. She asked and found out that Mrs. B, like herself, also suffered from knee arthritis. Mrs. B used to mountaineer very frequently in her younger days, so she believed that she was paying the price of overusing her knees.

Mrs. B prefers natural things, and that even applied to her choice of medical treatment for her aching knees. She had shunned from prolong use of anti-inflammatory or pain medications, and she was suspicious of injections of drugs into her knee cavities. But when she heard about the ACRFP treatment that Mrs. A had received, Mrs. B was tempted. When she saw how well Mr. A had recovered and bounced back, Mrs. B was confident that she herself could benefit from the ACRFP. Together Mrs. A and Mrs. B went to see Dr. Lyu, who performed the ACRFP on them on the same day in **May 2013**.

Chapter 9

The two of them followed the dos and don'ts exactly as directed by the case manager at the Knee Centre. They walk the 1.2-mile stretch from their community to the school every day, they temporarily stop going to the hot spring house so that they do not risk falling, and they do the daily rehab exercises.

Mrs. B also dances with a group in the morning where she met Mrs. C, whose gaits betrayed her knee pain. Mrs. B told Mrs. C everything about her experience with the ACRFP. Mrs. C went to see Dr. Lyu without hesitation. Fortunately for Mrs. C, Dr. Lyu began offering a new clinic in Taipei on March 19, 2014, when Taipei Tzu Chi Hospital inaugurated its own knee centre. There, Dr. Lyu performed the ACRFP on Mrs. C in **May 2014**. Around that time, Mr. A and Mrs. A and Mrs. B had their two- and one-year follow-up at the Taipei hospital as well. All three of them were satisfied with their progress.

About a year later, the four of them made a special request so they could have their annual follow-ups on the same day, so Mr. A, Mrs. A and Mrs. B, and Mrs. C had their three-, two-, and one-year follow-up together in May 2015. Mr. B and Mr. C, though not patients, went with them. It was more an excursion than a visit to the doctor. It was a joyous journey for the four patients because they have all regained their mobility, and it was a fun trip for Mr. B and Mr. C, too. They were happy to see the others feeling so well about themselves again.

It has been a nice retirement for all six of them.

Chapter 10 Evidence-Based Medicine Part II: Physician's Clinical Experiences

I was a resident surgeon in Taiwan from 1983 to 1987, an attending surgeon from 1987 to 1989, and trained in orthopaedics from 1989 to 1990 at Rush-Presbyterian-St. Lukes Medical Centre in Illinois, United States, Tübingen BG Unfallklinik, Germany, Geneva University Hospitals, and the Bern University Hospital, Switzerland.

Like many, if not all, newly minted surgeons, I returned to Taiwan in 1990 as an attending orthopaedic surgeon, fully confident that my surgery techniques would be able to solve all the ills of my patients. I got involved with arthroscopy, then just emerging, and delved into designing surgical techniques to fix sports injuries. At that time, I thought these seemed more exciting and more difficult than treating knee OA.

Like most orthopaedic surgeons, I was then of the opinion that there were only two ways to treat knee OA: total knee replacement for severe cases and pain management for less severe patients. While they are on pain medication, their knees are otherwise untreated, so their knees continue to deteriorate. As an orthopaedic surgeon, it is frustrating to be unable to provide active treatment when the knees are still relatively healthy. My helplessness left many patients on pain medication, waiting in agony, and allowing their knees to slowly go worse and worse. When the deterioration was bad enough to warrant surgery, the damaged knees are replaced with artificial prostheses.

All orthopaedic surgeons have probably experienced this feeling of helplessness. In fact, that helplessness has existed since ancient times, but mainstream modern medicine has so far not diminished that impuissance or substantively improved the treatment protocol.

Chapter 10

Trying to change this situation, I organised and established a research team for the study of osteoarthritis of the knee in 2002 and developed, step by step, the KHPO.

Nowadays, in an average year, I see 1200 new outpatients, do 250-300 knee replacements, and perform ACRFP on 750-900 knees. These numbers would have been higher if I had not curtailed the intake of my outpatients. I have intentionally lowered the number of patients in the clinic because I have been fully booked on my surgery calendar for many years, forcing my patients to wait 18 months or longer for the ACRFP. I have performed as many ACRFP procedures as I can, week after week, year after year. Still, the waiting line has only grown longer. Patients, lots of them, are in pain, they want relief, and they are willing to wait for the ACRFP so they can regain function, lose the pain, and keep their knees.

Patients deserve this minimally invasive procedure, and I am more than willing to help them. But there is a limit to the number of operations I can do in a week. My calendar slots have become a bottleneck that has kept the waiting line growing. I need other surgeons to help, and patients need other surgeons to help too.

Perhaps one day not too distant, knee OA will require only minimally invasive arthroscopic treatment instead of knee replacement. Who would have thought that AIDS and cancer are now viewed more as chronic and manageable than as acute and life-threatening that they once were?

Chapter 10

Orthopaedic surgeons who have experienced the ACRFP

To train more surgeons to become familiar with the ACRFP and the KHPO protocol, I have from time to time taught classes about the subject. Some orthopaedic surgeons from Taiwan, United Arab Emirates, Bangladesh, India, and China have taken these training courses, both in-class lecture and clinical. Below are some of their thoughts about the ACRFP.

1. **Dr. Yang Lin-Min,** attending physician (orthopaedics), Cheng Ching Hospital, Taichung, Taiwan. [Dr. Yang took the ACRFP clinical training course from March 12 to April 26, 2012.]

I heard about the ACRFP, but I did not believe the good results it had achieved. Now I have seen it firsthand, and I have to believe that ACRFP and its benefits are real. **It's just hard to believe that modern medicine, as advanced as it is, has continued to keep Dr. Lyu and his ACRFP out of mainstream treatment protocols.**

I am fortunate to have personally witnessed and experienced the wonders of the ACRFP. I have been unable to find words to fully express my gratitude to Dr. Lyu.

I intentionally divided my study in the ACRFP workshop into four sessions with two weeks between sessions. This way, I would be able to practice at my hospital what I had learned in the workshop. I wanted this experience to sink in and my expertise to improve.

Every orthopaedic surgeon has tried and believes that he or she can do arthroscopy. That's what I thought going into the ACRFP workshop, and I immediately realised how mistaken I had been about that when I saw Dr. Lyu do arthroscopy.

Arthroscopes, in Dr. Lyu's hands, mesmerised me. I was witnessing the performance of a master. How can arthroscopy be performed to such ex-

Chapter 10

cellence? I wondered, no, I marvelled. He also made the procedure appear so simple to me.

Again, I was wrong about that. When I went back to my hospital, I tried to apply what I had learned from Dr. Lyu. I quickly realised that everything that he had done so effortlessly was in fact quite difficult for me to do. I could hardly do even one procedure. There is more to the seemingly simple ACRFP than meets the eye. I decided to delve into it.

Now I have gained some basic proficiency in the ACRFP, but I know quite well that I have a very long way to go before I can reach Dr. Lyu's preeminent mastery of the art.

I have been most fortunate to have witnessed the efficacy of the ACRFP on knee OA, and I will use the procedure to help my patients.

I am deeply grateful to Dr. Lyu, and I hope to return to him for more training.

[A follow-up report from Dr. Yang on June 20, 2012:]

I recently treated a few more difficult arthroscopic cases:

- ACL avulsion fracture s/p ORIF with arthrofibrosis and knee stiffness. I used Dr. Lyu's method to perform the release, which helped the patient gradually regain range of motion.
- Gouty arthritis: I used a shaver to slowly clear whitish crystal disposition.
- Uni-K with medial side severe pain. Medial plica could be seen in arthroscope showing signs of inflammation. I removed the plica, and the pain went away. Just like magic.

Thank you, Dr. Lyu, for teaching me. I can now serve more patients.

Chapter 10

2. *Dr. Huang Jian-Rui*, attending physician (orthopaedics), Hoping Hospital, Taipei, Taiwan. [Dr. Huang took the ACRFP clinical training course from October 13, 2014 to January 27, 2015.]

In February 2014, at the invitation of Dr. Lin Jian-zhong, chief of orthopaedics at my hospital, Dr. Lyu came to our operating room to perform a teaching ACRFP surgery on an arthritic knee. I witnessed techniques that only a master surgeon could so deftly execute.

The operation was completed in less than 15 minutes. The operation was truly an eye opener for me. The patient, sorely in arthritic pains before the surgery, soon recovered and became pain-free. The result was also truly astonishing for me. **I had just witnessed a treatment that was not recognised in mainstream care protocol for knee OA, and I had also just witnessed a result that the mainstream care has been unable to deliver so far.**

Before this demonstration surgery, I had already heard Dr. Lyu talk at my hospital in a scholarly gathering about treating knee OA. His concept flew in the face of traditional way of thinking, and his concept turned my dated thinking about knee OA on its head. My old way of practice was stuck in a rut, and I wanted to learn this new technique from him at Dalin Tzu Chi Hospital.

My wish came true in October 2014. I first went to his clinic to observe. It was packed, but he carefully examined and patiently talked to each patient about their situation as if they were his family—I already learned something from him. It was past seven o'clock in the evening when he finished with the last patient of the day. The clinic closed ten solid hours after it had started. Dr. Lyu went on to answer my questions clearly and completely. He was not holding any little secrets back from me. He truly wanted to teach me. I was moved.

I also observed in his operating rooms. He carefully explained surgical techniques to me, and he clearly pointed out important details throughout the operation. His diligent teaching has helped me tremendously, and I have a better understanding and appreciation of the Knee Health Promotion Option.

Chapter 10

After each training session with Dr. Lyu, I would return to my hospital and resumed my responsibilities. I would carefully select a few suitable patients to receive the ACRFP. In preparation for each operation, I would meticulously and repeatedly go over in my mind every step that Dr. Lyu had taken during the procedure. Despite such efforts to get ready, in my first few attempts on the ACRFP in my own operating room, I had to spend more than an hour to complete the procedure, which Dr. Lyu routinely takes ten minutes to finish.

That did not discourage me. Instead, I kept thinking back, trying to isolate the problems, I watched the video teaching tapes on Dr. Lyu's website again and again, and I asked Dr. Lyu questions. My skills have gradually improved with each effort.

I have treated patients with ACRFP, and I am happy to report that some of them experienced dramatic improvements as if they had been reborn. Their excruciating knee pains suddenly disappeared. Some of them started walking without walking sticks, which they had not been able to do before the surgery. I witnessed those miracles with my own eyes. I cannot help admiring Dr. Lyu for his great contributions to the human race.

Today is the last day of my training with Dr. Lyu. I feel distinctly ambivalent. On the one hand, I am glad that I have completed this training course, but on the other hand, I don't feel like saying good-bye. I hope to come back for more training under Dr. Lyu, and I hope that I can use the techniques that I have learned here to help many patients. I shall not let Dr. Lyu down.

I would also like to thank the folks at the Joint Centre. They have taken great care of me and they have taught me much.

Chapter 10

3. ***Professor Liu You-Han***, MD, PhD in orthopaedics, the University of Tokyo, attending physician (orthopaedics), Hope Doctors Hospital, Miaoli, Taiwan. [Dr. Liu took the KHPO introductory course on January 23, 2010, the partial and total knee replacement workshop on February 27, 2010, and the ACRFP clinical training course from April 14 to May 6, 2010.]

Upon my arrival at Dalin Tzu Chi Hospital on January 23, 2010, my first impression of Dr. Lyu was that he had been mindful in arranging the training. He assembled physicians from family medicine, pathology, and immunology to teach us. The course was a highly systematic review [of knee OA], and it helped us refresh our memories of medial plica.

"Pannus" was by no means unfamiliar to us, but when we heard Dr. Lyu say "pannus-like tissues", we still could not suppress our curiosity. But when we heard "genu articularis muscle", our jaws dropped. "Wow, this stuff does exist."

When Dr. Lyu showed us all types of plicae and the damages they could cause, I was deeply ashamed of myself for knowing so little about medial plica, and what I thought I knew about it was quite misguided. He showed us PFJs [patellofemoral joints, or kneecaps] that had been severely worn out of shape by medial plica at locations that did not get in contact with cartilage. He showed us numerous real cases of such abrasion.

While training with Dr. Lyu, I was fortunate to have seen many patients of knee OA in his clinic and operating room being transformed from suffering to relief. Take the young female patient, I think it was the third case on the first day of training, for example. Her knee pain had made her wheelchair-bound when she went to see Dr. Lyu. After he removed her medial plica, she became totally pain-free. That's totally amazing.[This procedure was not arthroscopic resection, which does not have this efficacy. This procedure is the ACRFP.]

I saw how he conducted his clinic. He treated new patients warmly, patiently, and informatively. I was particularly struck by his patients returning for post-surgery follow-ups. Their warmth and gratitude towards Dr. Lyu was remarkable. They told him how much the operations had relieved their pain. Their relief was just amazing.

Chapter 10

I remember one old patient. He was from Miaoli. There was no joint space in his knee to speak of. The femur was kissing the tibia. But one year after Dr. Lyu's surgery, the space between the femur and the tibia returned. The knee space has opened up. I know that's unbelievable [in the minds of surgeons following conventional treatment guidelines], but that is the truth. I am curious if the cartilage in the old patient's knee has regenerated or what has grown back in that space. No matter. Even if he has gotten back fibrocartilage, that is good too. [The patient's pain is gone.]

Anyway, very impressive.

And that was not the only case of dramatic improvement that I witnessed at Dalin.

I know that, **as great as Dr. Lyu's treatment really is, he has some diehard doubters and detractors. To those people, I want to say, "Seeing is believing."**

Now some comments about Dr. Lyu.

I remember reading a paper a few years back. It said something to this effect: A TKR [total knee replacement] surgery takes about two hours. Only a genius or a quack does it faster. A genius fixes the knee and makes the patient feel better after surgery while a quack botched the knee.

A beautiful TKR, from the first incision to finishing the first-layer stitch, takes Dr. Lyu about 40 minutes. Clean, crisp, precise, and downright fast, it is so smooth and seems so effortless that it is beautiful. It is art.

His UKA [unicompartmental knee arthroplasty, partial knee replacement] and ACRFP are likewise impressive, precise, and fast.

Watching Dr. Lyu operate, I know that he has a well-thought-out plan for every surgery. Every cut and each hammer strike is exact and just so.

I may sound like I am bootlicking to Dr. Lyu, but I am not.

To be fair, I am not exactly a novice in knee surgery. In my practice, I perform TKR between 150 and 200 times a year, but I have not been able to do

Chapter 10

it as quickly and gracefully as Dr. Lyu. From him, I have learned something that I can use in my practice.

Though I started in surgery earlier than Dr. Lyu, his expertise and skills in this space are head and shoulders above mine. I can learn many things from him, and I am surely glad that I have met such a great teacher.

4. **Dr. Siddnarth Patel,** attending physician (orthopaedics), [Dr. Siddnarth took the KHPO clinical course from December 5 to December21, 2012.]

Respected Dr.Lyu SR,

I am very thankful to you to have given us this opportunity to come to Da-Lin and learn about the KHPO program including Uni-K and TKR surgery. It has been a great educational and cultural trip to Taiwan. Your Vision of KHPO is really great and I assure you that in the coming years it will be an internationally recognised treatment modality for knee OA.

Like Dr. Ponseti for CTEV, you will be Dr. Lyu for OA knee!

I personally believe that KHPO is tailored and made for Indian patients, as the routine lifestyle of Taiwanese people is very similar to that of Indians and **I have personally seen your long-term follow up patients who are completely satisfied and cured of OA knee**. This method will definitely be a success in India.

It is a beginning of a journey,

THE KHPO JOURNEY of: Seeing → Believing → Practicing

Most of my feelings have already been written by Dr. Amit in regards to our accommodation, education and especially your hospitality. **I have gained a lot of knowledge not only in ACRFP but also in Uni-K & TKR.** I thank you for your kindness in telling us all the tips and tricks in ACRFP, Uni-K and TKR. I also have to mention that our trip to The National Chung Cheng University was very helpful to us in understanding the pathology of knee OA.

I would like to personally thank your team especially Gefu, Kasma, Chia-Chi, Su-Mei, Ruby and Rachel and all the kind staffs of yours for the overwhelming love shown to us.

With this I promise to practice KHPO and spread awareness of KHPO and the actual pathology of knee OA that the world has still now not seen.

With this I ask for your blessings for me to practice KHPO and ACRFP in the correct manner. Also as mentioned by Amit, we would love to coauthor

Chapter 10

your work in our national orthopaedic Journal, after we have had our own set of cases.

This is just the beginning of a teacher-student relationship between us that will remain forever.

I wholeheartedly invite you and your family to stay and tour India with us. Also I promise to work hard to invite you as an international faculty for a conference/workshop.

I thank you for this past amazing 3-weeks.

Thank you!

Yours sincerely,

Dr. Siddharth Patel
Ashirvad Hospital
Gujarat, India

Chapter 10

5. ***Dr. Chowdhury Iqoal Mahmud,*** attending physician (orthopaedics),. [Dr. Mahmud took the KHPO clinical course from November 14 to November 23, 2012.]

Dear Dr. Lyu,

I would like to express my heartfelt thanks and gratitude for giving me the opportunity to attend your KHPO fellowship program. It's an honour for me to acquire knowledge from you and also sharing my working experience with you. I think I have acquired enough knowledge and information from you. So that I can start treating my OA patients when I go back to my country.

In my opinion, your concept of treating OA knee will have a big impact in our country regarding the treatment of OA knee. I am sure millions of OA patients will be benefited from KHPO program. I have no doubt that your method of treatment of OA patients will be accepted worldwide in very near future.

I have immensely enjoyed my fellowship here in Dalin Tzu-Chi Hospital. All the supporting staffs have been extremely kind and supportive. I would recommend this fellowship program to other orthopaedic surgeons.

I wish your good health and success, so that you can pursue your dream.

Thanks to all the supporting staffs and thank you very much. God bless you.

Kind regards

Sincerely yours
Dr. Chowdhury Iqoal Mahmud
MBBS, FRCS, MCh Orth
Assistant Professor of Orthopaedics
BIRDEM Hospital
Dhaka, Bangladesh

Chapter 10

6. **Dr. Jonaed Hakim,** resident (orthopaedics),. [Dr. Hakim took the KHPO clinical course from November14 to November 23, 2012.]

Dear Sir,

"When you know a thing, to hold that – you know it, and when you don't know a thing, to allow that you don't know it – this is knowledge" – Confucius.
Thank you sir, for enlightening me with such knowledge. Being a resident in orthopaedic surgery, having young eyes full of dream, and tender mind to flourish, this fellowship will give me the opportunity to think about osteoarthritis of the knee, as well as, of pain related to the knee. You have shown how beautifully you manage these problems by KHPO and gave patients a big relief. No doubt, it's a new idea, a new journey. And sir, you are traveling this journey with faith, courage and wisdom. "…Every tree trunk contains the homes of insects, every leaf can be the nest of dewdrops. Every road has the shoe prints of travellers, or perhaps the print of their feet. But the trail of each shoe print or footprint is eventually covered and obliterated by the wind and dust. To be a 'traveler', one can only go forward all alone." – Xiang Yang (Lin Chi-Yang)
I believe this journey of yours will see its peak very soon.
And you are not alone, sir, we are with you.
Finally, thanks to you, your team and all the beautiful Taiwanese people, who made the days here a very wonderful and memorable days of my life.

Thank you all

Dr. JONAED HAKIM

Residence of Orthopaedics
BIRDEM Hospital
Dhaka, Bangladesh

Chapter 11 Evidence-Based Medicine Part III: The Best Scientific Evidence

While on a rushing train in Bavaria, Germany in 2000, I made this bold hypothesis:

"The repeated contact between the medial plica and the medial femoral condyle during knee motion causes the 'medial abrasion phenomenon', which is an important cause for the gradual degeneration of articular cartilage."

The ACRFP appears simple, but it is effective, and it is based on solid science. My collaborators and I have published 12 papers on every aspect of this set of arthroscopic procedures for knee OA. The papers are listed below.

Chapter 11

My research team

Shaw-Ruey Lyu, MD, PhD

    Director, Joint Centre, Dalin Tzu-Chi General Hospital, Chiayi, Taiwan

De-Shin Liu, PhD, Professor

    Advanced Institute of Manufacturing for High-tech Innovations and Department of Mechanical Engineering, National Chung Cheng University, Chiayi, Taiwan

Wen-Hsiu Hsieh, PhD, Professor

    Advanced Institute of Manufacturing for High-tech Innovations and Department of Mechanical Engineering, National Chung Cheng University, Chiayi, Taiwan

Lai-Kwan Chau, PhD, Professor

    Department of Chemistry and Biochemistry, National Chung Cheng University, Chiayi, Taiwan

Hwai-Shi Wang, PhD, Professor

    Department of Anatomy, National Yang-Ming University, Taipei, Taiwan

Yung-Chih Kuo, PhD, Professor

    Department of Chemical Engineering, National Chung Cheng University, Chiayi, Taiwan

Hong-Tzong Yau, PhD, Professor

    Advanced Institute of Manufacturing for High-tech Innovations and Department of Mechanical Engineering, National Chung Cheng University, Chiayi, Taiwan

Chapter 11

Our Research Projects

Explore the pathogenesis of knee OA
    Clinical and epidemiological study (SR Lyu)
    Anatomical and biomolecular study (SR Lyu, HS Wang)
    Finite-element model study (SR Lyu, DS Liu)

Conceptualise novel treatment modality
    Development of KHPO (SR Lyu)
    Repair the damaged cartilage (SR Lyu, YC Kuo)
    Biomechanics analysis of cartilage tissue (SR Lyu, WH Hsieh)
    Culture and cryopreservation of chondrocyte (SR Lyu, WH Hsieh)
    Bioengineering of cartilage (SR Lyu, YC Kuo)

Promote the new concept
    Virtual reality teaching system for arthroscopic surgery (SR Lyu, HT Yau)
    Study for community needs (SR Lyu)
    Combine to health promotion system (SR Lyu)

This theory and its resulting surgical techniques under the KHPO protocol have helped several thousand patients of knee OA loss pain, regain mobility, and regain function. If those satisfied patients of ours are any indication of the usefulness of the KHPO protocol, we believe the following is true too: This seemingly simple theory of medial abrasion phenomenon as a cause of cartilage damage and its clinical applications (ACRFP under the KHPO protocol), as laid out in the following 12 papers, will gradually change how knee osteoarthritis will be treated in mainstream medicine.

Under conventional treatment protocols, "Degenerative Arthritis (Osteoarthritis)" has been a catch-all diagnosis that practitioners assign to knee arthritis when they are not sure of its cause. The term "Degenerative Arthritis (Osteoarthritis)" has led to two misconceptions: (1) Knee OA is an unavoidable consequence of ageing, and therefore (2)

Chapter 11

knee OA has no cure and that the best that medicine has to offer the patient is pain management.
"Degenerative Arthritis (Osteoarthritis)" has become a term of irresponsible medicine, a term that all responsible physicians will not use. As you will see in the following points, there is **a better diagnosis: Medial Abrasion Syndrome**.

In the past, conventional medicine could not explain the process of cartilage degeneration in "knee osteoarthritis". Now, our papers have proved that the "medial abrasion phenomenon" can fully account for that cartilage degeneration process.

In the past, conventional medicine could not explain the various clinical symptoms of "knee osteoarthritis". Now, our papers have provided that the "Medial Abrasion Syndrome" fully accounts for all these symptoms.

Treating patients who are older than 40 years old complaining about knee pains, physicians should take "Medial Abrasion Syndrome" into account. Not doing so may lead to a misdiagnosis and the patients' disease may deteriorate.

"Knee osteoarthritis" is no longer a disease for which there is no cure. If a diagnosis of "Medial Abrasion Syndrome" caused by medial abrasion phenomenon can be made early enough, there is a chance that the disease can be cured.

In conventional medicine, most patients who are older than 40 years old complaint of knee pains, tightness, joint swelling, and reduced mobility have often led to the diagnosis of "knee osteoarthritis". These symptoms in fact indicate that the patients might suffering from the "Medial Abrasion Syndrome", which is caused by the medial abrasion phenomenon. The syndrome can be effectively treated with the Knee Health Promotion Option, the KHPO.

Chapter 11

Published papers

Here are the 12 papers directly related to our core theory of medial abrasion phenomenon as a cause of knee OA and its clinical application that my collaborators and I have published so far.

1. Knee health promotion option for knee osteoarthritis: a preliminary report of a concept of multidisciplinary management. *Healthy Aging Research*, 2015, 4:34.
2. Role of medial abrasion phenomenon in the pathogenesis of knee osteoarthritis. *Medical Hypotheses*, 85 (2015): 207-211.
3. Medial Abrasion Syndrome: A Neglected Cause of Knee Pain in Middle and Old Age. *Medicine*, April 2015, Volume 94, Issue 16, p e736.
4. Relationship between medial plica and medial femoral condyle—a three-dimensional dynamic finite element model. *Clinical Biomechanics*, Volume 28, Issues 9–10, November–December 2013, Pages 1000–1005.
5. Matrix Metalloproteases and Tissue Inhibitors of Metalloproteinases in Medial Plica and Pannus-like Tissue Contribute to Knee Osteoarthritis Progression. *PLoS ONE*, 8(11): e79662.
6. Arthroscopic cartilage regeneration facilitating procedure for osteoarthritic knee. *BMC MusculoskeletalDisorders*, 2012, 13:226.
7. Matrix metalloprotease-3 expression in medial plica and pannus-like tissue in knees from patients with medial compartment osteoarthritis. *Histopathology*, 2011, 58(4), 593-600.
8. Medial plica in patients with knee osteoarthritis: a histomorphological study, *Knee surgery, sports traumatology, arthroscopy: official journal of the ESSKA*, 2010 Jun., 18(6):769-76.
9. Arthroscopic medial release for medial compartment osteoarthritis of the knee, *J Bone Joint Surg Br*, September, 2008, Vol 90-B, issue 9, Pages 1186-1192.
10. Relationship of medial plica and medial femoral condyle during flexion. *Clinical Biomechanics*, 2007, Volume 22, Issue 9, Pages 1013-1016.

Chapter 11

11. Mechanical strength of mediopatellar plica - The influence of its fiber content. *Clinical Biomechanics*, October 2006, Volume 21, Issue 8, Pages 860-863.
12. Medial plicae and degeneration of the medial femoral condyle. *Arthroscopy*, 2006, 22(1):17-26.

The following article is a summary of most of the findings in the papers above.

Knee Health Promotion Option for Osteoarthritic Knee: Cartilage Regeneration is Possible

(Full Text: http://www.intechopen.com/books/osteoarthritis-diagnosis-treatment-and-surgery/knee-health-promotion-option-for-osteoarthritic-knee-cartilage-regeneration-is-possible)

Chapter 11

Other papers published under our research projects:

1. Measuring transport properties of cell membranes by a PDMS microfluidic device with controllability over changing rate of extracellular solution. *Sensors and Actuators B: Chemical*, 197(2014): 28-34.
2. Quantification of Tumor Necrosis Factor-α and Matrix Metalloproteinases-3 in Synovial Fluid by Fiber-Optic Particle Plasmon Resonance Sensor. *Analyst*, 2013 Aug 21;138(16):4599-606. doi: 10.1039/c3an00276d.
3. Experience-based virtual training system for knee arthroscopic inspection, *BioMedical EngineeringOnLine*, 2013, 12:63.
4. Forced-convective vitrification with liquid cryogens. *Cryobiology*, 66-3 (2013):318-325.
5. Cryopreserved chondrocytes in porous biomaterials with surface elastin and poly-l-lysine for cartilage regeneration. *Colloids and Surfaces B: Biointerfaces*, 103(2013):304–309.
6. Application of albumin-grafted scaffolds to promote neocartilage formation. *Colloids and Surfaces B: Biointerfaces*, 91(2012):296–301.
7. Integration of fiber optic-particle plasmon resonance biosensor with microfluidic chip. *Analytica Chimica Acta*,2011, 697(1-2):75–82.
8. Fiber-optic particle plasmon resonance sensor for detection of interleukin-1β in synovial fluids. *Biosensors and Bioelectronics*,2010, 26(3): 1036-1042.
9. Study of cryopreservation of articular chondrocytes using the Taguchi method. *Cryobiology*,2010, 60(2):165-76.
10. Cryopreservation and biophysical properties of articular cartilage chondrocytes.*Cryobiology*,2005, 51(3):330-8.

Chapter 12 The Making of an Ideal KHPO Surgeon

The ACRFP under the KHPO is an effective treatment for many patients who suffer from knee OA, and I make this claim based on thousands of cases, behind each of which is a real person—a former patient of knee OA—who has benefited from the KHPO. This KHPO efficacy is reproducible among patients, and there are far more patients of knee OA who need the KHPO service than I can possibly serve.

The knee OA sufferers everywhere need many more—hundreds of thousands more—KHPO surgeons, but at this time, there are very few surgeons in the world who are willing (to take a pay cut) and able (have the technical expertise) to become a KHPO surgeon.

What is in KHPO for the surgeon? I can answer in one sentence. You get the great satisfaction knowing that you have truly served an unmet medical need and your patients thank you for that.

Let me outline the requisite qualifications of an ideal KHPO surgeon.

Chapter 12

Knowledge set

Whenever something is new,
  people say it is not true.

As time goes on and it is proven to be true,
  people say it is not important.

As time goes on and it is proven to be important,
  people say it is not new anymore !

Voltaire, 1694-1778

Belief propels action. I hope that I have conveyed in this book sufficient information and evidence to convince orthopaedic surgeons that the KHPO is at least worth their time to explore, if only for the sake of their patients' knees.

Preconceived conventional notions about knee OA (Table 4) that medical schools and orthopaedics academies have instilled deeply into the minds of orthopaedic surgeons are the primary and formidable roadblocks that have prevented new treatments from receiving mainstream acceptance.

Our KHPO program has compiled ample data (X-rays, arthroscopic images, and others)—backed by feedback from thousands of patients—to debunk those conventional notions. Despite such evidence, however, conventional treatments for knee OA, like old habits, die hard.

Therefore, the first step for a conventional surgeon to transform into a KHPO surgeon is for him or her to, let me not mince words, wipe the slate clean.

Chapter 12

I understand that this is asking a lot, and I understand that only the most courageous surgeons will be able to make such a huge commitment to serve patients. Often this means for the surgeon to do less of an established procedure (TKR) to which he or she is accustomed and quite proficient at performing, and to do more of a strange procedure (ACRFP) which he or she never heard of, much less learned, in med school, residency, or clinical practice.

I know all this because I myself was once such a conventional surgeon, a very well established one at that. Still, I made the transition, and it has been a most gratifying journey ever since. I feel overjoyed and fulfilled whenever I hear the great relief that my surgeries have brought to my patients with OA knees—relief that Uni-K and TKR have been unable to deliver. If you asked me, I would answer unequivocally, "Yes, I'd gladly take this journey again if the chance were offered me," if I may borrow a few words from the Nobel laureate Bertrand Russell.

It is understandable that the more entrenched and established a conventional surgeon is, the more difficult it would be for her or him to accept KHPO and scale back the utilisation of knee replacement that has served her or him so well for so long. For those surgeons, I shall only remind them that **all** their TKR patients have lost their knees, and **most** of my ACRFP patients have kept their own knees.

Chapter 12

Table 4. Knowledge about knee OA

Conventional Concept	KHPO Concept
Knee OA has unknown etiology	MAP* is a main etiologic factor for knee OA
Knee OA is inexorable and irreversible	With ACRFP, knee OA could be halted and reversed
Damaged cartilage cannot regenerate	Damaged cartilage could regenerate
Knee OA can not be cured	Knee OA could be cured if treated in time
Knee replacement is the unavoidable ultimate treatment	Knee OA's degenerative course could be arrested and reversed, and knee replacement could be avoided

* MAP = Medial abrasion phenomenon

Chapter 12

The skill set

Most orthopaedic surgeons specialising in arthroplasty do not perform arthroscopy, and vice versa. An ideal KHPO surgeon, however, should master both arthroplasty and arthroscopy and utilise the one or the other without prejudice. Which procedure is ultimately chosen for a patient is determined mainly by the patient's situation and not by the surgeon's surgical preference.

ACRFP is an arthroscopic surgical procedure that is technique- and experience-intensive. It takes years for a surgeon under supervised learning to become fully proficient in the ACRFP.

A well-designed training program will provide the needed theoretical and clinical training for an orthopaedic surgeon to become a good KHPO surgeon. We provide one such training program:

> **Professional Learning Course for KHPO:**
> http://www.joint.idv.tw/plc.en/

Chapter 12

Mind set

The training for orthopaedic surgeons in a sense looks like that for carpenters. However, an ideal KHPO surgeon should have both the dextrous hands of a consummate carpenter and the compassionate mind of a good gardener:

Table 5. The KHPO surgeon as a gardener

KHPO Surgeon	Gardener
Teach patients the right ways of knee care	Teach the right principle of gardening
Perform ACRFP in time to provide a more hospitable environment in the knee cavity for cartilage to regrow	Soil preparation, weeding, and keeping bugs away
Knee care after ACRFP in the hope that cartilage will regenerate	Care for the garden correctly in the hope that it will regenerate
Arthroplasty if condition worsens	If the condition worsens, dig out everything and replant

Moreover, an ideal KHPO surgeon must hold the patient's best interest above all other interests—not even his or her own financial interest should get in the way and influence his or her choice of procedure to perform on the patient.

If financial considerations figure dominantly in your career, then the KHPO may not score the highest in your calculations. However, if serving an unmet medical need, serving your patients extremely well, and during that process making a respectable and quite comfortable living makes you happy, then I believe that you have what it takes mentally to become a KHPO surgeon.

Appendix

Appendix 1:   She helps make ACRFP work so well
- A complete story of a desperate retired teacher and her recovering knees

My name is H. Y. Wang. Today is April 26, 2015.

About twenty years ago, when I was 46, at the height of my career, I had arthroscopy on not one but both knees. That was followed by more than **ten years of hyaluronic acid injections**. The efficacy of the injections gradually diminished with time, and my knees were in pain more often than not. My doctor advised knee replacement, and I reluctantly agreed. But I got cold feet before the scheduled surgery.

When I was 59, I could not stand for too long, could not squat down, and could not walk with decent stability. I often lost control of my legs when I took the stairs up or down. The excruciating pains impelled me to see doctors all over the place. Almost all of them recommended some version of this: "Manage and put up with the pain till you're 65 or till your knees deteriorate completely. Then you get a knee replacement."

At that time I was almost constantly in pain, whether I was standing, sitting, walking, sleeping, or turning in bed. A good night's sleep was a luxury for me, and quality of life was just a pie in the sky. It was a huge challenge to limp my way through a single day. There was no way that I could survive with any dignity for six more years [when I turn 65].

I could not exercise, I was just about housebound, and I was sleep deprived. Imagine to go on like that. If I had had to wait years for my knees to worsen enough to qualify for knee replacement, my body would have worsened right along with them. If my body is shot, what is the point of getting new artificial knees?

Appendix

Platelet-rich plasma, or PRP, finally became available when I was 60. I eagerly got PRP shots on both of my knees for three months, setting me back NT$90,000 (US$3,000). It was wonderful as the pains eased off, but only for nine months. Then I began to **suffer the consequence of PRP injections**: I could not sit for long; after getting off a bus my knees would sometimes lock up, and I could not take even a step; I had to rely on a walking stick to keep from falling; and I had excruciating pains that made me cry.

I could not go on like that, so I tried rehabilitation. It did not help. "My knees were tied", so I could only consent to **steroid treatments**. Steroids were a bad idea because my knees hurt even more. I suspect that was a consequence of following PRP shots with steroids.

All right, no steroids, so I tried PRP and hyaluronic acid injections all over again, much like recycling. The same treatments got me only the same result, and I watched another US$3,300 drained away.

The doctor suggested that I try partial knee replacement. I was scared to death, but I refused to give up hope. I tried traditional Chinese medicine, acupuncture, and all manners of folklore treatments. As these experiments, or straws grabbing, were ongoing, my knees undoubtedly continued to wear away. Several months and much money later, my knees still hurt. The traditional Chinese medicine did not work, either.

I could only return to my orthopaedic surgeon who told me that all the cartilage in my knee was totally worn and there was abrasion lesions on my kneecap. The damage was so severe that he would not recommend **autologous mesenchymal stem cell transplantation or chondrogenesis**. He could only recommend total knee replacement. He told me, as if to console me, that new artificial knees could last 25 years.

I doubted that. My father-in-law had had an unsatisfied knee replacement before. Moreover, after having knee replacement surgery, my own father was injured in an automobile accident. The artificial knee protruded so badly that he could not have a corrective surgery. He was committed to bed until he withered to his death. Knee replacement did not appear to be a

Appendix

panacea. Knee replacement did not instil much confidence or comfort in me.

I met a woman at a clinic. She had had knee replacement five years earlier. Her artificial knees were inflamed and loosened because of her severe osteoporosis. Her case drove home the point that knee replacement is a path of no return. Knee replacements should never, never be taken lightly. They should be done only after all avenues of possible remedy have been exhausted.

And I thought I had tried everything, and nothing had seemed to help. Things really did not look good. I was desperate. I was scared to death. Who could save me?

I was grabbing straws. Any straws would seem better than nothing, but I still tried to tell myself to be rational. At this critical moment, a good friend told me about Dr. Shaw-Ruey Lyu, about the arthroscopic cartilage regeneration facilitating procedure, ACRFP, that he had developed, and about how many knee OA sufferers had benefited. It all sounded good, but was it too good to be true? I cautioned myself not to raise my hope. I already had had too many dashed hope.

I watched every teaching tape on Dalin Tzu Chi Hospital's website about the ACRFP, and I read every posting on Dr. Lyu's blog and every article about the philosophy, approach, facility, staff, and everything else that I could find, and then his Chinese book came out, and I read that too. I read the book again and again, and I took careful notes.

I attended several workshops that he offered. After each event, I stayed behind to ask him questions. He was always patient and helpful in answering them. I made an appointment for his clinic. He looked at my X-rays and checked my knees. I was a nervous wreck because he was looking at my condition, and he was telling me specifically about my knees, not generally about any knee. I felt that this clinic was truly different from all the ones that I had had before; I felt hope in this one. He was empathetic, and he cared. He did not want me to have knee replacements when they were not absolutely necessary, and fortunately for me, they were not.

Appendix

Suddenly, all the years' false hopes, real disappointments, fear, despair, and all the pent-up desperation found an outlet, and I cried in his clinic. I shed happy tears. I felt hope, and I knew that I would no longer be helpless. I got on Dr. Lyu's surgery calendar for arthroscopic cartilage regeneration facilitating procedure, or ACRFP.

While waiting for the operation, I strictly followed his advice to do the three exercises (leg raise, knee hug, and press knee) every day, to not carry heavy things, to avoid taking the stairs, and to avoid biking in order not to exacerbate my knee OA.

Finally it was my turn for the arthroscopic surgery in February 2015. I had spinal anesthesia, so I was fully alert during the entire surgery. I stared at the monitor that showed the surgery live as Dr. Lyu explained to me what he was doing, such as arthroscopic loose body removal, arthroscopic synovectomy, and arthroscopic medial release. I felt entirely at ease knowing that I was in good hands.

After the surgery, I was off the bed and walking later that same day. I have since then most diligently carried out the daily rehab regimen that he prescribed. It is this diligence to stick to the rehab and to his list of the dos and don'ts that has enabled me to recover rapidly. The tearing pain that had constantly accompanied me for so long before the ACRFP is now completely gone.

Now I feel only some occasional swelling and, when I do the knee hug, some tightness. I keep telling myself to stick to the rehab no matter what. These are temporary pains, and persistent rehab exercises will make them go away soon. When I occasionally got carried away and used my knees too much, I would do the knee raise and use heat pads to soothe the pain. These are must dos.

My knee pains are gone. I am living proof of the wonders of the KHPO treatment. Cartilage does regenerate, but it takes time. It grows back slowly but surely.

Appendix

Here is my advice to the people who are suffering from the same kind of knee pain that I did.

Be a good patient. A good doctor cannot do it alone. It takes a team to get the job done, and the team includes the patient. The doctor has fixed what was wrong, and it is time that the patient takes over, does the simple rehab routine every day, and follow the dos and don'ts without fail.

Without the patient's post-surgery cooperation and efforts, all the hard work that the doctor has done will be futile. Only when both parties do their bit can the KHPO, or any other treatment, have any chance of succeeding.

I am grateful to Dr. Lyu. Two months after the surgery, I am able to do house chores normally. I walk half an hour a day, and everything is quickly going back to normal. I am getting my life back.

Generally, Dr. Lyu's surgery patients return for followup visits at one, three, and six months after the surgery. After that they return on anniversaries. In my first followup clinic, I saw an old woman who was there for her three-year followup. She showed people in the room how well she was able to stand, squat, jump, and raise her legs. She was back to normal, and she is older than me. She gave me a shot of hope in the arm. Though I am not quite there, I am quite sure that I will be as good as she.

I would like to thank Tzu Chi Foundation for its patient-centric approach to medicine. With its support, physicians like Dr. Lyu can conduct research and practice medicine that is best for the patient, though not necessarily best for its bottom line.

If Dr. Lyu had practiced medicine for profit first and foremost, he would have recommended knee replacements to me. After all, knee replacement is the mainstream treatment for knees like mine, and doing knee replacement is more profitable. Fortunately for me, he has chosen to be different, to do what he believes is right for his conscience, his intellectual challenge, and his patients.

Appendix

I am glad that I had second thought and I got cold feet on knee replacement all those years. For once procrastination was a good thing: It helped me find Dr. Lyu. With the good things that I have found out about the KHPO, you do not have to put it off any more. Ask your doctor if the AMR or the ACRFP is right for your knee.

I know I would not hesitate to spend money on such a wonderful treatment, but I actually spent less, much less, than I would have spent on a total knee replacement. I keep my knees. I am happy, and I hope you can be, too.

H. Y. Wang's update on December 13, 2015:

On February 26, 2015, Dr. Lyu performed the ACRFP on both of my right and left knees, which were suffering from grade IV and III knee OA, respectively.

Though confident of the benefits of the ACRFP, I have nonetheless experienced discomfort, pain, relief, doubt, and bliss—a physical and emotional rollercoaster ride—on my journey of recovery from the surgery.

But I have never wavered in my resolve to follow the four-times-a-day rehab exercises even though they are at times painful to do. The pain is part of the recovery. I would rather deal with this temporary pain than allow contracture to form and ruin my knees again. Now there is much less pain during my rehab exercises and much more fun and joy in my everyday activities. I am glad that, despite the pains, I have persisted in following Dr. Lyu's directions on rehab exercises.

I am now able to do most things comfortably, without pain. I take walks, volunteer, travel, cook for my family—I am enjoying life. If I stand for *too* long, my knees still hurt a little. But I am still recovering, and I believe that, with diligent rehab, I will be able to stand longer and longer as time goes on.

Appendix

I believe that my recovery and enjoyment are possible because of two things: One is Dr. Lyu's ACRFP surgery that removed the cause of my knee OA, and the other is my strict adherence to the rehab exercises every day. My recovery is unfolding exactly as he has planned for me, and that includes the pain of overcoming contractures.

I am sharing my experience in the hope that my fellow knee OA sufferers can also benefit. It just feels wonderful to know that my OA knee pains are all gone and that my occasional minor pains are just signs of recovery from surgery, which will eventually disappear.

Best wishes to you.

Milestones of my recovery after the ACRFP:

1. February 26, 2015, the day of surgery: Got off the bed to stand on a walker at 17:00, 20:00, and 22:00. Walked in the room.

2. The day after surgery: Got out of my bed and walked five times. Started doing the rehab exercises.

3. Two days after surgery: Discharged. Sat in the front seat of our car with legs elevated on support. My husband carried me up the stairs because our apartment building did not have an elevator.

4. Seven days after surgery: Dr. Lyu removed the suture. Checking how much I could bend my knees, he knew that I had done the rehab exercises as he had ordered. I cooked and did the laundry at home.

5. Fourteen days after surgery: Hot pads made the knee bending exercise easier. I bent all the way in. It hurt so much that tears came out, but it was worth every drop of it. I could bend my knees much easier the next day.

6. At the one-month recall, Dr. Lyu reminded me that scars were forming inside me and that I should diligently do the rehab exer-

Appendix

cises despite the pain, which he pointed out would be more intense than before. He suggested that for three months I should not take a bus or sit for too long with my knees bent. I should walk more but on flat surfaces without overtiring myself.

7. Two months after surgery, I was able to do all my housework and shopping. I took a day trip. I no longer felt any OA knee pains.

8. On May 16, 2015, almost three months after surgery, the left knee hardly hurt anymore. The right knee, which was stage IV knee OA, hurt occasionally, but even it was much better. I took the city bus for the first time. I went to places freely for family gatherings. I had a camping trip in June. Sitting or standing too long still caused pain, a good reminder to do rehab exercises diligently.

9. Six months after surgery, I started volunteering, and I walked at least 30 minutes a day.

10. One day in the ninth month post-op, I took a day tour to a reservoir and a flower expo during which I sat, climbed, and walked—too much. I was out from 6:00am to 9:00pm that day. I clearly did too much. I had to take hot baths, use hot pads, and do rehab exercises extra hard for five days before I recovered from the indulgence.

11. In my 10th month now, though my knees still hurt slightly if I stand for too long, I am a very happy volunteer and grandmother. If you are considering getting the ACRFP or recovering from it, have confidence in the program. It has helped me a great deal.

Thank you, Dr. Lyu, for saving my knees and saving me from my OA knee misery.

Appendix

Appendix 2:   The three rehabilitation exercises under the KHPO

Like toothbrushing for oral hygiene, these rehabilitation exercises are recommended to be performed lifelong for the health of your knee.

Always sit in a comfortable and stable chair with a back!

Appendix

"Leg Raise" for quadriceps strengthening

Objective: to strengthen and keep the endurance of your thigh muscle

Leg Raise

Four sessions each day: morning, lunchtime, dinnertime, and bedtime

For each session:

1. Raise right leg **off** the chair. Keep the knee extended and the ankle flexed toward your body.
2. Raise the leg to the height of the butt
3. Hold 10 seconds.
4. Repeat the above 10 times.
5. Switch to the left leg and do the same.

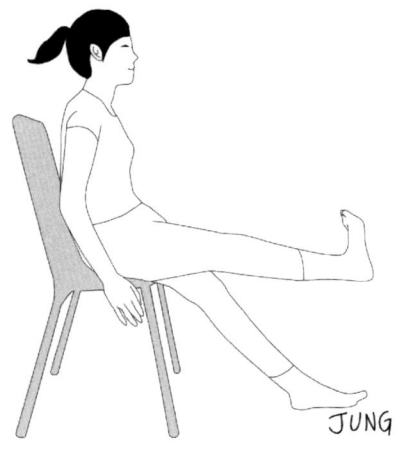

Appendix

"Knee Hug" for anterior soft tissue stretching

Objective: to maintain appropriate tension between cartilage

Knee Hug

Four sessions each day: morning, lunchtime, dinnertime, and bedtime

After each session of leg raise:

1. Grab the right ankle with both palms, slowly pull the ankle as close to your body as possible.
2. Hold as long as you could.
3. Switch to the left leg and do the same.

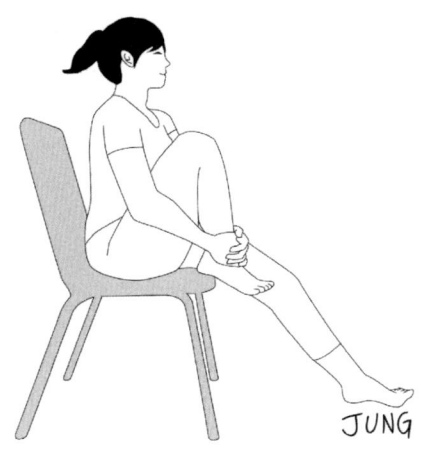

Appendix

"Press Knee" for posterior soft tissue stretching

Objective: to maintain appropriate tension between cartilage

Press Knee

Four sessions each day: morning, lunchtime, dinnertime, and bedtime

1. Put the right heel on a stool in front of you.
2. Extend the right knee.
3. With both palms on the right knee, steadily press down.
4. Hold 10 seconds.
5. Repeat 10 times.
6. Switch to the left leg and do the same.

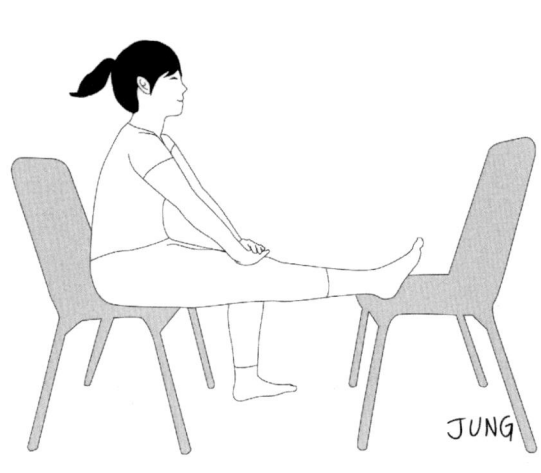

Appendix

Appendix 3:   Activities to enjoy or to avoid before and during the first post-operative year of ACRFP

To facilitate cartilage regeneration, strict rules about engaging in appropriate daily activities and exercises should be followed during the first post-operative year. The rationale for this precaution is to avoid repeated bending of the knee that might produce shearing forces harmful to cartilage regeneration.

In general, activities and exercises requiring repeated knee bending (> 50 degrees according to our research) are regarded as harmful to the knee before and during the first post-operative year of ACRFP. Based on this principle, Table 6 shows some activities that are suitable for or harmful to the knee before and during the first post-operative year of ACRFP.

Table 6. Suitable and harmful activities before and during the first post-operative year of ACRFP

Suitable Activities	Harmful Activities
Walking	Climbing up or down stairs
Jogging	Mountaineering
Golfing	Squatting (e.g. Gardening)
Freestyle swimming	Bicycling
Butterfly swimming	Breaststroke swimming

About the Author

Biography

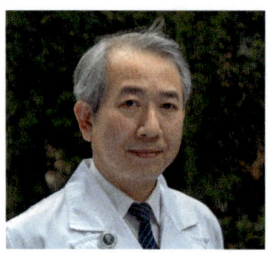

Born on August 9, 1958, in a small town of Hsinchu, Taiwan, Dr. Shaw-Ruey Lyu is a renowned knee surgeon who has brought conventional treatment of knee osteoarthritis into a new era. Having witnessed first-hand the hope that his father brought to his patients as a family doctor, SR decided at the age of 6 that he wanted to work in the medical field. After graduation from National Yang Ming University, he was a resident surgeon in Taiwan from 1983 to 1987, an attending surgeon from 1987 to 1989, and trained in orthopaedics from 1989 to 1990 at Rush-Presbyterian-St. Lukes Medical Centre in Illinois, United States, Tübingen BG Unfallklinik, Germany, Geneva University Hospitals, and the Bern University Hospital, Switzerland.

Like most orthopaedic surgeons, he was then of the opinion that there were only two ways to treat knee OA: total knee replacement for severe cases and pain management for less severe patients. While they are on pain medication, their knees continue to deteriorate. As a surgeon, it is frustrating to be unable to provide active treatment when the knees are still relatively healthy. His helplessness left many patients on pain medication, waiting in agony, and allowing their knees to slowly go worse and worse. In fact, that helplessness has existed since ancient times, but mainstream modern medicine has so far not diminished that impuissance or substantively improved the treatment protocol.

He decided to pursue the cause of knee OA in 2002. His pursuit has eventually led to a dozen research papers, the recognition of the terms "Medial Abrasion Syndrome (MAS)", the "Arthroscopic Medial Release (AMR)", the "Arthroscopic Cartilage Regeneration Facilitating Procedure" (ACRFP), and the "Knee Health Promotion Option" (KHPO). More importantly, he has used these treatments to relieve thousands of knee OA sufferers of their debilitating pains. A vast majority of them have kept their knees, have been pain-free, have regained function, and have resumed their lives.

Made in the USA
Middletown, DE
09 September 2016